# Revitalize
# Your Life
# After 50

# Jack LaLanne

# Revitalize Your Life After 50

## Improve Your Looks, Your Health and Your Sex Life

HASTINGS HOUSE *Book Publishers*
Mamaroneck, NY 10543

Library of Congress Catalog Card Number 93-078853

ISBN 0-8038-9356-6

Printed in the United States of America

10   9   8   7   6   5   4   3   2

*To my wife Elaine "La La" and to all the people who have stood by and believed in me all these years.*

# Acknowledgments

My wife Elaine for her countless hours at the computer editing this book.

Gale Shemwell Rudolph Ph.D., a good friend and a consultant in nutrition and food science, for helping to keep me informed and up to date.

Carolyn Katzin, M.S. in nutrition, for her suggestions.

My daughter, Dr. Yvonne LaLanne, D.C., and her husband, Dr. Mark Rubenstein, M.D., for their recommendations.

Lance Carter, our office computer expert, who not only taught Elaine to use the computer, but for his time reading and rereading the manuscript.

Brenda Rodrigues, our secretary, for being there when we needed her.

Richie Ornstein for suggesting that I do this book.

Hy Steirman and Hastings House for wanting to publish it.

# Contents

# Foreword

As I look back and reflect on the sixty-five years in my profession of Physical Culture, I arrive at this conclusion about life: Age is only a number, and with the mind and the body, anything is possible if you make it happen.

You may think that miracles were performed only in biblical times. I beg to differ. Thousands of miracles are happening every day. I believe it's a miracle if an overweight, out-of-shape person loses 50 pounds and reshapes his or her body. If people double their strength and endurance and look and feel years younger, to me that is a miracle. When their attitude changes and they are happier than they have felt in years, that is a modern miracle.

If you will incorporate the common sense, nutrition, and exercise outline I give you in this book, I promise you too can experience a miracle. As my mother often used to say, "God helps those that help themselves." I hope and pray you will make the small effort and help yourself to a new life. Remember again, **anything in life is possible,** just make it happen.

Let's get started.

Healthfully and enthusiastically,

Jack LaLanne

# Jack LaLanne Feats

Age 40: Swam the length of the San Francisco Golden Gate Bridge under water with 140 pounds of equipment, including two air tanks . . . an undisputed world record.

Age 41: Swam from Alcatraz to Fisherman's Wharf in San Francisco wearing handcuffs.

Age 42: Set a record of 1,033 pushups in 23 minutes on "You Asked for It" TV show with Art Baker.

Age 43: Swam the treacherous Golden Gate Channel, towing a 2,500-pound cabin cruiser. This involved fighting the cold, swift ocean currents that made the 6½-mile swim a test of strength and endurance.

Age 44: Maneuvered a paddleboard 30 miles, nine and one-half hours nonstop from the Farallon Islands to the San Francisco shore.

Age 45: Completed 1,000 pushups and 1,000 chinups in 1 hour and 22 minutes.

Age 60: Swam from Alcatraz Island to Fisherman's Wharf, handcuffed, shackled, and towing a 1,000-pound boat.

Age 61: Swam the length of the Golden Gate underwater, handcuffed, shackled, and towing a 2,000-pound boat against treacherous tides.

Age 62:    Commemorating the "Spirit of '76," swam one mile in Long Beach Harbor, handcuffed, shackled, and towing thirteen boats (representing the original thirteen colonies) containing seventy-six people.

Age 65:    In Lake Ashinoko, Tokyo, Japan—handcuffed and shackled, towed sixty-five boats filled with 6,500 pounds of Louisiana Pacific wood pulp.

Age 66:    In North Miami, Florida—towed ten boats filled with seventy-seven people for over a mile in less than an hour.

Age 70:    Handcuffed, shackled, and fighting strong winds and currents, towed seventy boats with seventy people from the Queen's Way Bridge in Long Beach Harbor to the Queen Mary, 1½ miles.

Jack LaLanne's birthdate is September 26, 1914.

# Revitalize Your Life After 50

## Chapter 1

# Fiftysomething: You're Halfway There!

I once heard a memorable comment in a play. The question was asked, "How old do you have to be to reach old age?" The answer was, "Old age is someone twenty years older than yourself."

So whether you're 50, 60, or 70—old age is always 20 years away. It's a healthy attitude to have. I feel that you have three ages: your chronological age (your actual age), your physical age (how you feel today), and your psychological age (how you feel mentally). The old saying, "You're only as old as you feel," is absolutely true. I know I'm eightysomething and I feel the same as when I was thirtysomething. So what have I been doing the last fifty years? The same thing I've been doing all my life, looking after myself, and that's my advice to you.

But how about those of you who haven't been looking after yourselves? You're constantly tired, suffer from hundreds of little aches and pains, don't enjoy a happy love life, and have generally become a couch potato. In other words, "Your get up and go has got up and went." Your self-esteem has dwindled, you hate the way you look, your house has become your tomb, you feel sick but you enjoy being sick, and you don't feel like cooking anymore. You're in a panic, the give-up stage of life. You think your youth has gone and you're "over the hill," even though the rat race has been won, the kids are grown, the mortgage paid up, and your house is just the way you want it. Well, it's time to break down the aging process and recharge your battery. Let's see how we can start revitalizing your life to improve your looks, your health, and even your sex life.

The fifties, sixties, and seventies are simply stages of life. It wasn't a crisis when you made the change from infant to adolescent to teenager, then to adult. Why then should it be a crisis to become 50, 60, 70, or even 80. I believe that age is just a series of numbers. When I turned 80, I realized that I was just half of 160 and when I make that, I'll be half of 320. I want you to stick around and find out!

Like wine, you should be able to improve with age. Nothing in medical science says the body falls apart after 50. With the new national interest in healthy nutrition, the latest advances in medicine, and the campaign to cut down on smoking, the external forces are at work trying to help you. There are some things you must do for yourself, however. The truth is, too many individuals have been brainwashed to accept the over-the-hill blues. They think it's time to "pig out," stop exercising, and take it easy.

If you think about it, Winston Churchill was 65 at the start of World War II when he became Britain's Prime Minister, President Franklin D. Roosevelt was 59 when Pearl Harbor was attacked and he led America to victory. Grandma Moses didn't start painting until age 76 and she lived to be 101. Sophocles wrote *Oedipus Rex*, one of the greatest plays of literature, at age 90.

In more current times, the Senior Olympics and the

Senior Golf Tour are becoming more and more popular. Ronald Reagan was president well into his 70's, Colonel Sanders began his career at 65, Dr. Spangler was running marathons in his nineties. Then there's the vivacious "Dancing Grannies" who are in their fifties, sixties, and seventies. How about the man who bungee jumped at age 100? I could go on and on. Why are you any different?

There is no distinct dividing line between the young and the old. Some folks die at 40 and they bury them at 60. Have you been busy dying instead of living? Why surrender to a myth that becomes a self-fulfilling prophecy, i.e., if you think you're old, you *are* old? The corollary is, if you think you're young, then you *are* young. I staunchly believe that thoughts are things.

By surrendering, we let ourselves go. We let the sags and bulges appear on our bodies as well as in our minds. Sags and bulges make women and men look older than they are. Thus, they feel older.

Try this little test: Place a 10-pound rock or 10 pounds of flour in a tote bag. Better yet, go to the market and get 10 pounds of fat and carry it around with you for a few minutes. Heavy, isn't it? Now, if that was 10 or 20 pounds of extra body weight you were carrying around, aren't you helping to speed up the aging process? Obesity can lead to many complications, including diabetes, heart problems, and strokes. One of the worst diseases for some is "mirror-itis": When you look in the mirror you get sick.

I enjoy my life more every day. The French have a wonderful expression, "Joie de vivre!" which means "The joy of life." A bundle of joy popped into my life when I was almost 50. I became a father again! Most of the good things in my life have borne fruit in my mature years. I took up golf at 50 and at age 72 I shot my age and eventually got down to a 4 handicap.

If you have fallen into the age trap of no exercise and exceeding the feed limit, start fighting the problem with a positive approach. Learn to know yourself, to love yourself. Look in the mirror, make a mental image of how you want to look, and then see yourself that way. Be cognizant of this mental image constantly. When you feel like indulging in that extra dessert, call up that mental image. Think of carrying that tote bag of fat around with you. Make short-term goals for yourself. A fitness program without goals is like a ship without a rudder. Set a course and follow it through. See the end result in your mind's eye.

Remember, you are only halfway there. The feeling of being "over the hill" can affect your current life only if you let it, or it can be a happy time during your prime years for building happier years to come. I'm sure you've heard the saying, "The only thing constant in life is change." So if you are sick and tired of being sick and tired, make yourself happy and make a change. Start to control your destiny by getting rid of old concepts. Remember, age is only a number. Science has shown us that more and more people are living to be over 100. This is not a time of great deterioration if you invest a little effort in energizing your vigor and vitality. Along with proper nutrition, better medical and personal body care, you will be revitalizing your life.

# Chapter 2

# Just Do It!

Once upon a time there were two fat, contented middle-aged frogs, Mike and Ike. They lived on a grassy rise of ground beside a farm lane and spent their days snaring flies and croaking happily. Mike and Ike had it made, and they knew it.

As the living got better they got fatter and a bit more awkward. One day while reaching for a fly, Ike lost his balance. He landed in the bottom of a wagon rut with a loud *Humph!* There he remained all night, unable to leap back up to his grassy knoll.

The next morning Mike called to his partner, "Jump out, jump out!" Fat old Ike shook his head forlornly and cried, "I can't, I can't. I'm too old and too fat. I'm over the hill!" Several days went by and Ike was beginning to get uncomfortable in the rut. For one thing his appetite was killing him. There weren't many flies in the rut, Mike had them all to himself.

Being a frog, Ike lost weight fast, and with it strength from the lack of exercise. As it is in middle age, Ike quit figuring how to get out of the rut. He just hunched there despairing, recalling the good life he'd had. In a way he regretted the blind gluttony with which he'd eaten flies, burying his youth in ounces and ounces of frog fat. A big frog tear rolled down his wan green cheek.

Suddenly Ike felt a rumbling. Glancing over his shoulder, he gasped. A big farm wagon with two huge wheels was rolling relentlessly down the rut, ready to crush Ike to death. Closer and closer it came. Ike tried to leap out of the way but couldn't move. "Is this," he thought, "my end? And so young!" The wagon rolled on. Ike had experienced dreams like this when he'd eaten one fly too many. This wasn't a dream. He trained again, croaking in terror. The wheel was coming close, almost upon him.

He had to do something. He gave one last tremendous leap and landed safely on the bank. It happened so suddenly it amazed even him. He had lifted himself out of the rut. The wheel rumbled over the spot where he'd just been. His life was spared. Mike was cheering loudly, saying, "You did it Ike! You did it! How in the world did you do it?" Ike answered, "I had to!"

The moral is similar to the one I propose to you as we tackle this "over the hill" business. When he *had* to do something the frog discovered that he could. So can you! When he realized what it was like to live in a rut he never wanted to go back. You won't either. We can do things if we have to.

There are many kinds of ruts in life and many ways of falling into them. And there are ways of getting out. Most ruts are states of mind, and getting out doesn't always require desperation leaps. The second half of our lives, to some of us, is the worst rut to face. However, we don't have to do anything drastic to get out of it. It's easier for us than for the frog. We just choose to make a few changes.

The first step is to change your thinking. Like the frog, leap into life. Quit accepting the rut you're in. Learn to fight for your life. I'll show you and help you but you'll have to help yourself. This book is designed just for that purpose. We're going to discuss proper foods and exercises for vigorous living and for your physical well-being.

As it's often been said, the rest of your life is the best of your life. I'm reaching for your hand now to help you reassess your attitude on living and jump into the happiest, healthiest, most productive years you will ever have.

I believe in miracles. I won't accept that miracles stopped happening 2,000 years ago. That unconquerable human spirit of body and mind hasn't changed in twenty centuries. Add to that the know-how of modern science and nothing is impossible.

I can even teach you to lift 1,000 pounds. Impossible you say? It might be, if you didn't know how. We'll start by having you lift 1 pound; the next day that might be too easy so you'll lift 2 pounds. Then 5, then 10. If you lift 10 pounds 100 times you're lifting 1,000 pounds, aren't you? It's the same with life's problems: one step at a time.

Maybe you're 30 pounds overweight right now. You think of those 30 pounds and the days of dieting trying to lose them. The task seems Herculean. You're discouraged before you start, so you don't start. Thirty pounds then become 35 and so on up the scale.

Nothing is Herculean if you tackle it a pound at a time and a day at a time. Mix in a song, some laughs, plus a vision of the result. The next thing you know, you're dropping 5 pounds, then 10. Tell yourself, "Mine is not a hopeless case." Repeat it with confidence. Once your mind is made up and you've established a mindset, the doing will be simple.

You're skeptical? Consider the story of Henry S., who at age 49 became impotent. He feared he would lose his wife, who was 35. His doctor could find no medical reason for his loss of sexual powers and recommended that Henry, who was 20 pounds overweight, trim down. That brought him to me. We got Henry in condition by exercising, improving his diet, and adding vitamin supplements. Then it was mostly a matter of getting Henry to convince himself that he wasn't over the hill. As he felt better, proud of his physique rather than ashamed of it, self-confidence returned. His virility hadn't gone, it had only been inhibited.

How about the alcoholic secretary. Fortysomething, unmarried, who wrote me after leaving a recovery program. She was sober for the moment, but admitted life held little promise. After reading her letter on my television show, there was an avalanche of response, offering reassurance and workable daily suggestions. I outlined a regimen of nutrition and exercise to improve her physical well-being. Things began to happen fast. For the first time in her life she could see tangible results in something. Looking better and feeling better about herself, she started to meet and mix with other people and to recognize that they also had problems and frustrations. Gradually despair vanished as she lifted herself out of the terrible rut of alcoholism.

My Beat-the-Fifties program is really quite simple, as simple as a drink of water. But why water? More than 70 percent of our bodies is fluid (newborn babies 85 percent; no wonder their skin is so smooth). As the years pass, somehow, we don't drink nearly the amount of good, clean water we should. Little wonder then that when a person reaches 40 or 50 the skin often appears dry and dehydrated. Water keeps your cells fluid, helps curb your appetite, and assists you in keeping the weight off because it flushes the salt from your body (as you know, salt retains water). Water also flushes and cleanses the kidneys, liver, and spleen along with aiding the peristaltic action that promotes regularity. It thus stands to reason that drinking water should help slow the aging process.

I urge all adults to drink eight to ten glasses of water daily. If water isn't accessible, you're not as likely to drink your daily requirement. I suggest that you keep a bottle near you, whether it be in the gym, car, or your office. If the taste of water is too bland, squeeze in a little lemon juice for taste and vitamin C.

The program I have for you requires a little more than drinking enough water every day. We're going to work your body but we have to prepare it before it's ready for action. Number one, it's advisable to get a medical checkup with your health professional. If you are able to begin an exercise program, that's a plus right there. Don't procrastinate. Start immediately. Repeat the words of the expression you have probably heard many times: "Today is the first day of the rest of my life."

As soon as you open your eyes and before you roll out of bed, count your blessings, don't complain, be thankful for what you have, and don't dwell on things you don't have. Now, simply do bed stretches. Reach out with your arms, legs, fingers, toes and stretch. Make your body as long as you can. Reach and stretch. Now take a couple of big deep breaths to fill those lungs. Inhale through your nose and exhale through your mouth. (Never inhale and exhale at the same time!)

Watch animals when they awaken. What is the first thing they do? Stretch. I'm convinced, if you stretch properly you will be healthier and look more youthful. You will also be more flexible in your movements.

As we age, many people complain about their muscles becoming stiff. It's not the muscles that become stiff, it's the ligaments and tendons that connect the muscles to the bones. They are like rubber bands. If they are not used they become brittle and lose their flexibility.

You have 640 muscles and all these have ligaments and tendons, and when you stretch, it takes muscle action to stretch them. Your posture improves, helping your internal organs to function better, along with increasing circulation. Stretching will also pep you up when you are tired from sitting or lying around. Stretch several times a day but check with your doctor before starting an exercise or diet program.

Here are some added stretches to get the day started:

**Ceiling Stretch:** Stand with your feet a shoulder width apart. Lift your arms over your head, palms up, stretch as if you were trying to touch the ceiling or the sky. Count to 10, relax, and count to 10 again.

**Side to Side Stretch:** Begin just as you would the Ceiling Stretch. While reaching for the ceiling, keep your feet planted solidly on the floor. Now, slowly and smoothly, bend at the waist from one side to the other. Count to 10 on each side. Relax and count to 10 again. Do not overstretch and do not use jerky movements.

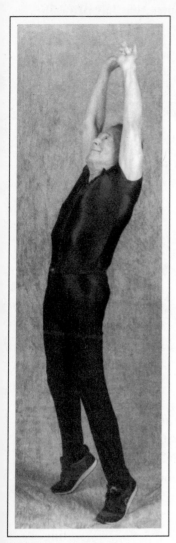

**Ceiling stretch**

**Side to side stretch**

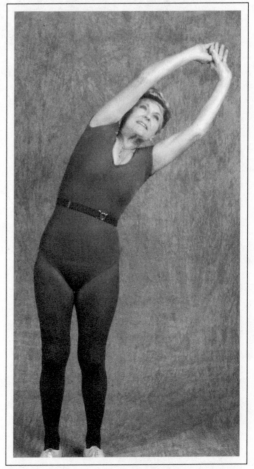

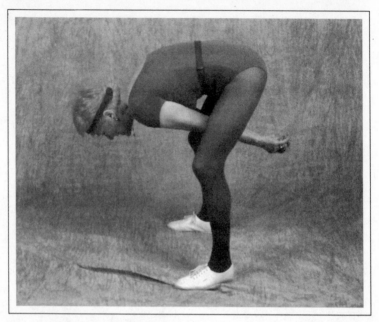

**Through the legs stretch**

**Through the Legs Stretch:** Plant your feet a shoulder width apart. Bend forward at the waist, knees slightly bent to take the strain off the back. Bring the hands through the legs, attempting to touch the floor and wall behind you. Hold for a count of 10, relax, repeat and hold for a count of 10.

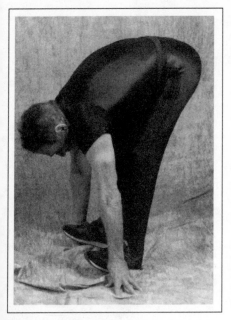 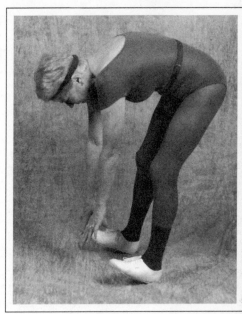

**Hamstring stretch**

**Hamstring Stretch:** Place your feet a shoulder width apart. Bend forward at the waist, knees slightly bent. Allow your hands to drop down in front of your feet, as though trying to touch the floor. Now, lift the toes off the floor. Hold for a count of 2. Feel those hamstrings stretch.

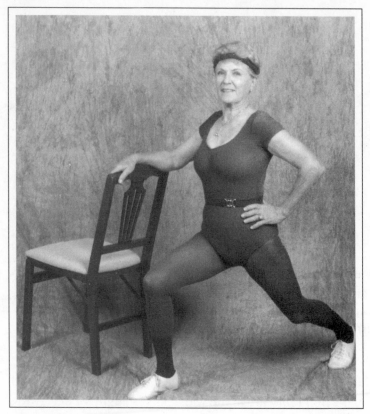

**Leg lunge stretch**

**Leg Lunge Stretch:** Stand erect, hand on hips (or on a chair for balance). Lunge forward (similar to a fencing pose). Hold for a count of 5. Step back and lunge forward on the opposite leg and hold for a count of 5. These can be done lunging to the side as well.

Now that you have got your blood circulating with some stretching, cast out all traces of yesterday's blues. Think about the good food you will be eating today, the new exercises you are going to try, and the things you mean to accomplish. Don't let any thoughts derail your optimism. Take inventory. Sit down with a pencil and paper and list all the liabilities you keep associating with your life. Beside them, list your assets, every skill, talent, bit of property, bank account, qualification, and characteristic that can work in your favor. See what you have going for you. I bet the pluses outnumber the negatives. Once you see this you can start disposing of some of your worries and concerns. Perhaps life isn't as bad as you thought it to be. The very fact that you are able to exercise is a plus. Look on the positive side. Even if you are in a wheelchair there are some parts of your body you can move.

Don't let your body deteriorate, don't procrastinate; let's begin to revitalize your body now. Like the frog that jumped out of the rut because he *had* to, jump out of your rut because you *want* to, not because you have to.

## Chapter 3

# So Who's Perfect?

The devastating thing about thinking you are over the hill is the self-defeating attitude that nothing can be done about it. I think I've heard all the excuses, including: "I get out of breath so easily, I can't exercise," "I'm so thin now I would be afraid to lose any more," "I'm a fatty and I'll always be a fatty, so I've decided to accept myself the way I am," "I've got an arthritic shoulder," "I'm too old," or "I've got a bad back."

So who's perfect? Well, I'll tell you. *No one!*

As a physical culturist for over sixty years, I've met thousands of men and women in all stages of physical condition. But I've yet to see a perfect body.

I have worked daily on my own body, mind, and personality for over a half century with nearly every nutritional and exercise tool available and I'm far from satisfied. But I am happy because I've made great improvements.

Who's perfect? The Hollywood stars? Not really, yet they refuse to let secondary defects age them prematurely or deter them from fruitful lives. Clark Gable, the great symbol of handsome masculinity, had oversized ears and every one knew it. Beautiful Elizabeth Taylor has frequently had to overcome serious illnesses. How many leading men are short or wear toupees? How many female stars fight battles with weight or depression?

That's the point. People like this refuse to be held back by handicaps.

Lord Byron had epilepsy. So did Julius Caesar, who surmounted this defect to conquer the world. Chopin composed great music though he had tuberculosis. Robert Louis Stevenson wrote some of his greatest literature despite the same illness. Admiral Nelson won his historic naval battle at Trafalgar though he had but one eye and one arm. Franklin D. Roosevelt, despite being crippled by polio, traveled by wheelchair through twelve years as President of the United States. Beethoven was deaf, Stephen Foster an alcoholic and Abraham Lincoln a victim of depression. Even Florence Nightingale, the great symbol of unselfish nursing, was a sickly woman.

No one is perfect. I remember a man in his forties, with one leg, who came to my conditioning studio fifty years ago to improve himself. He was Vic Burgeron, owner of the famous restaurant chain Trader Vic's. Few people realize that Academy Award–winning star Jack Palance had been a bomber pilot in World War II. His face suffered severe burns when his plane crashed. Plastic surgery restored his face, but he had difficulty facing people. A psychologist suggested he take up acting to overcome his shyness. The rest is history.

I too have a handicap. In my last year at Berkeley High School in California, I underwent a serious operation on my right knee as a result of a football injury. The doctor said I probably would never walk again. I was on crutches for months. As time went on I decided I was not only going to walk but also recover completely. I found the steepest hill in Berkeley and made up my mind that one day I would make it to the top. Each day I could walk a little farther than I did the day before and after several months I finally made it to the top. That was 1933.

During World War II, I wanted to join the service but I was 4F because I was unable to do a full squat. However, I kept trying to join some branch of the armed forces. A friend was enlisting in the Navy so I tagged along. As I was going through the line I did handstands, push-ups, and many of my hand-balancing tricks. As luck would have it, I wasn't asked to do a full squat and I was accepted. The examining doctor was the surgeon who had operated on my knee.

At age 68 I was hit head-on in my car by a truck that went out of control. My good left knee went into the dashboard, and I had to have another operation. So you see, we all have defects of one kind or another.

My wife, Elaine, has also overcome injuries. One evening she was in her car waiting for the stoplight to change when a bus lost its brakes and hit her from behind. The impact ruptured the gas tank and sent her skidding into traffic from the Hollywood Bowl. She sustained a severe whiplash and a wrenched right side. For years she was in pain but persisted in her exercises and therapy. Today at almost 70 she says she's going on 19.

None of us will be 20 again. Maybe we have stocky bodies, or extra long bodies, weak eyes, stubborn hair, big ears, or long noses. We needn't expect to be Venus or Adonis, but we can concentrate on making ourselves look attractive. A woman in her eighties can't expect to look like a girl of 18 again but she can be a beautiful 80-year-old.

So you're 50, 60, 70, or 80. I strongly feel that with a little attention, exercise, and proper diet you can feel youthful again.

A good example of improvement is a fellow named Louie, who came to my gym in Oakland, California, when he was in his seventies. He was tired all the time, had poor eating habits, and was extremely overweight. He could hardly push up a 25-pound dumbbell. After working out for several months he was pressing 100-pound dumbbells. He had as good results, or better, at his age, as any young person. In fact, many in the sports-medicine profession are finding that people from 50 to 95 are getting the same results from their exercises as their young counterparts. Proving it is never too late to get in shape.

Let's get down to some specifics. Here are some exercises that are ideal for you because they can be done while you sit in a chair watching television. Those of you who are currently working out at a health spa, have a personal trainer, or home exercise equipment, can use these exercises to supplement your workouts.

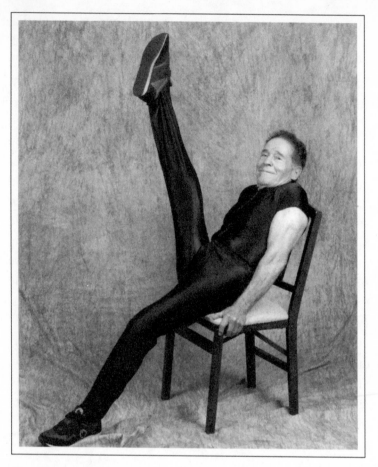

**Single straight leg lift**

**Straight Leg Lifts:** Sit forward on the edge of the chair, shoulders solidly against the back, gripping the sides of the seat with both hands. Now, with your legs straight, lift the right leg as high as possible and then the left leg, alternating right and left. Start with a count of 4 and work up to a count of 10 or 20. As you become more proficient, make little fast movements like a flutter kick. For those of you

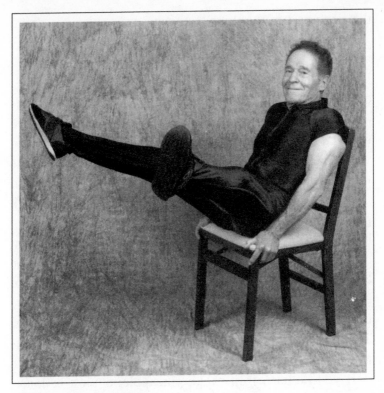

**Two straight legs lift**

who are even more advanced, lift both legs together up and down. This is beneficial for the lower abdomen, the hip flexors, and the muscles in front of your thighs.

**Leg Crosses:** This is a more advanced exercise. In the same position as above, lift both legs so that they are parallel to the floor. Cross and recross your legs. The better shape you are in the higher you hold your legs. When you cross your legs it helps develop the inner part of the thigh. When you bring your legs out to the side, it helps develop the outer part of the thigh. Leg crosses are also beneficial for the lower part of the abdomen.

If you're hungry after this, here's a dish that is delicious, offers a good vitamin balance, has lots of carbohydrates and protein, and is low in calories. We need to eat from five to seven fruits and vegetables every day, so I am suggesting vegetable or fruit salads. I'm going to suggest only the ingredients and you be the creator. For the vegetable salad I'd like you to try at least eight or ten of the following: dark green lettuce, red cabbage, bean sprouts, chopped tomato, broccoli, celery, bell peppers, jicama, carrots, cauliflower, cucumber, raw mushrooms, and garbanzo beans. You can also add hard-boiled egg whites, water-packed tuna, or even sardines to your salad. For a salad dressing use olive or canola oil with lemon or vinegar and herb seasonings. The utility of this salad lies in the fact that you may eat it as a complete lunch or in lesser quantity, as your dinner salad.

If you prefer a fruit salad, pineapple, apples, bananas, oranges, grapes, pears, peaches, apricots, berries, papaya, and mangoes are great. Top it off with a little nonfat yogurt.

These few suggestions will help beat the over-the-hill blues and fill you up, not out.

As I've said over and over on my television shows, "Exercise is a body normalizer, the food you eat today is walking and talking tomorrow."

## Chapter 4

# What Is Fitness?

Webster's dictionary describes fitness in several ways: "The state of being fitted; to be adjusted to the shape intended; to suit or be suitable; to be adapted; preparation." Like trying to define "love," it's impossible to come up with a definition that applies to everyone.

To me it's waking up in the morning with no aches or pains, a song in your heart, and a smile on your face. You work all day and still have the energy to do the things your mind wants to, when you want to.

I believe fitness is a balance between the mind and the body. In ancient Greek and Roman times the great athletes were the great scholars. They believed that the mind and the body went hand in hand. I believe you can't separate the mind and the body, what affects one affects the other. President John F. Kennedy once said, "Physical fitness is not only one of the most important keys to a healthy body, it is the basis of dynamic and creative intellectual activity. The relationship between the soundness of the body and the activities of the mind is subtle and complex. Much is not yet understood. But we do know what the Greeks knew: that intelligence and skill can only function at the peak of their capacity when the body is healthy and strong; and that hardy spirits and tough minds usually inhabit sound bodies."

When your mind says to you "jump," can you jump? When your mind says to you "run," can you run? Who's in charge, you or your body? *You* should be in charge.

As people get older and slack off on exercise and nutrition, they find they can't do the things they used to do, such as walk or run as fast, dance as long, or stay up as late. Now that's where fitness comes in. You can improve your strength, endurance, reflexes, and your overall condition by exchanging a few bad habits for a few good habits. I want to help you do the things you used to do. I want to help you to help yourself reverse the aging process. When this is accomplished your self-esteem goes up, your immune system is better, and you can cope with emergencies more readily because you have reserve energy to recoup faster.

Fitness is being prepared. It is an insurance policy, it's like having money in a savings account, it's there when you need it. It's the fountain of youth.

Being fit is unique to each of us, because each of us is unique in this great universe. Just as there are no two grains of sand alike or two leaves alike, so it is with us, there are no two bodies alike. Everyone is capable of achieving a level of fitness that is right for that person. You, and you alone, are responsible for your fitness, no one else can do it for you. However, you must want to become fit. We go through this life only once and we have only one body to take with us, so let's make the best of it. Everyone in the neighborhood of 50 or over would do well to run a personal check on what he or she is doing to promote fitness. Am I getting enough rest? Am I eating the right foods? Do I have a hobby that really relieves nervous pressures of my life? Am I exercising and building reserves of energy I need for true fitness? All of us should build that reserve just as we put money in the bank for the day we'll need it.

When we take care of our body it takes care of us, both physically and mentally. A fit body makes us feel better and look better, it makes us have more pride and discipline in ourselves.

One of my golden rules for complete fitness is: Make out a program of exercise that fits your needs. Work out vigorously at least three or four times a week at home or in a gym and on the other days do some stretching and/or fast walking. I'd like to see you do something every day so that you will rise above temptation and won't let yourself get out of the exercise habit. You eat every day, you sleep every day, you brush your teeth every day; I believe your body was made to move and that you should do some form of exercise every day. Change your program every two to three weeks because when a muscle gets used to doing the same thing it isn't challenged anymore. A muscle needs to be challenged to improve. Make exercise a habit for the rest of your life.

When I pioneered physical fitness with my daily TV shows, I received thousands and thousands of thank-you letters. I shouldn't have been thanked, my viewers should have thanked themselves because they are the ones who did the work. All I did was give them the tools. The point is, don't just sit there, do something! Fitness is the maximum you!

# Chapter 5

# Can You Change Your Life After 50?

I'm as vain as any man in his fifties, sixties, seventies, or even eighties, which is one compelling reason for working out daily to help keep my body as lean, muscular, and youthful appearing as possible. I am delighted (as you will be) when people remark, "You don't look your age."

In reality, I shouldn't have lived to age 50. Certainly not to become the father of a healthy, bouncing boy when I was almost 50. I was a tiny, sickly baby at birth whom my parents despaired of bringing through my teens. One serious illness after another threatened to cut me down before I finished high school. My father, an example of total surrender to bad health practices, was dead before he was 50.

When I reached 15 I did something radical. I changed my outlook on life and my way of living. It's something I suggest you do, even if you're 50 or over. I turned to the foods and habits that would stop the deterioration of mind and body and started a daily program of building against the years. I've told that story many times, but in case you haven't heard it, here it is again.

By the age of 15, I was a junk food junkie, a sugarholic. I had boils, pimples, arch supports, and glasses. I was weak, sick, and troublesome. Even the girls used to beat me up. I was so sick that I had to drop out of school for six months. It was during this time that a neighbor, Mrs. Joy, suggested to my mother that she take me to a health lecture in Oakland. My mother forced me to go. Not only was I inspired, but it changed my life completely. The lecturer, Paul Bragg, said that I could be reborn again, meaning that if I obeyed nature's laws, improved my eating habits, and exercised, I could change my body. I stopped eating white flour and white sugar products and joined the local YMCA. I was inspired! In fact, I was a strict vegetarian for six years.

My goal was to have a healthy body and play sports. I was almost 16 when I bought *Gray's Anatomy* and all through high school read it, re-read, and re-read it from cover to cover. (Many of my doctor friends have since told me that it was the most boring book they've ever read.) I was fascinated because it was going to help me fulfill my dream. I wanted to be an outstanding athlete and have a symmetrical, Mr. America type of body, along with physical stamina, strength, and endurance. I knew the workings of the muscles (myology) and bones (osteology) of the human body probably as well or better than most doctors and set out to make up for lost time and accomplish my goal.

I became the captain of our high school football team, and Amateur Athletic Union (AAU) state wrestling champion. I sold dates, nuts, honey, and other health foods to my friends and preached nutrition to my classmates. I set up a gym in my backyard with barbells and dumb-bells and began to design my own equipment. While still in high school, I had firemen and policemen working out in my backyard. They were my "guinea pigs." I would put them on specific individual programs of nutri-tion and exercise and month after month kept records of their progress. As time rolled by I knew exactly what to prescribe for the overweight, underweight, the old and the young. I had to learn by trial and error. It was sim-ilar to getting a Ph.D. in kinesiology (the study of the mechanics of human movement). Many of my class-mates shunned and resented me. They all thought that I was nuts.

I attended college with the aim of going into medicine but decided I wanted to help people before they got sick. In 1936 there were no places one could go to work out with weights other than boxing and wrestling gyms, which were called "sweat boxes." I wanted people to work out in a nice atmosphere—rugs on the floor, mirrors on the ceilings and walls, plenty of plants, clean glass-block showers, steam baths, and health foods. So I opened just such a place, with a health food store on the first floor and the gym on the second. It was at 409 15th Street in downtown Oakland and I paid $45 a month rent.

People made fun of me, saying there was some nut, a muscleman who was charging money to exercise. Doctors were saying "Don't go to that Jack LaLanne's, you'll get musclebound."

I went to the local high schools in a tight T-shirt and talked to the skinny kids and the fat kids about working out and eating right. I had to sell their parents on the idea. The kids got such great results that the parents started coming too. Several of those kids, Charles McCarl, Jack Schwarting, Norman Marks, Bruce Young, and Barrett Pierce, all went on to become physicians. All of them are over 70, in good shape, and continue to exercise daily.

To keep my clients interested, I would invent a piece of equipment; that's how the first pulley-machine using cables came into being. I also invented the first weight selector, leg extension machine, and many other pieces of equipment. I would barter for help and give memberships for expertise. Jack Palmer was a pattern maker who made patterns for my equipment. Russ Warner did all of my photographic work. In those days I never thought to patent anything and now those same concepts are used all over the world. I am still in touch with the people I have just mentioned and many more who helped me get started. I am so very fortunate to have them as my friends.

I continued to study, and graduated from chiropractic college. However, by that time I was working with M.D.s and due to conflicts between the chiropractors and M.D.s at the time, I kept my degree to myself.

By the time 1951 rolled around television was in its infancy. Because of my background I was asked to do a television show on nutrition and exercise. Eventually I had to sponsor myself. I sold only products that I believed in and subsequently developed the first powdered energy drink, which I called Instant Breakfast. The show later was syndicated nationwide and ran for over thirty-five years.

You can change your life too. Make your objective fitness. Anything you do will bring some improvement. In other words, anything is better than nothing. I made the important change during my midteens. My wife, Elaine, made the change in her thirties. Others don't make the change until their forties, fifties, sixties, up to their seventies. Some even wait until their eighties or nineties. The point is, it's never too late. So why wait?

Paul Summer of the National Center for Health Statistics prepared the following information on the major killing and crippling diseases in the United States. In 1990–91, there were 3,264,000 victims of mental and emotional disorders; 20,536,000 with diseases of the heart and circulatory system; 22,680,000 with hearing impairments.

The National Institute of Alcoholism informed us that Dr. Tom Harford's most recent National Health Interview Survey indicated there were 7,972,000 adults afflicted with the disease of alcoholism.

In the United States today almost one billion work days a year are lost through disability or chronic disease. Too many of these statistics grow out of the aches and pains from lack of physical activity.

I'm an idealist who will go to any length to help people go through life happier, healthier, more attractive, and successful. But I am also a realist. I know it isn't easy to take oneself in hand, despite rewards that are like an answer to our dreams.

I am positive that most victims of the fear of old age have already tried other positive teaching programs and lost interest somewhere along the way, sliding into the physical and mental state in which they now find themselves. Let's start to slide out right now with a simple little exercise.

Many of my birthday feats have to do with swimming. I believe swimming is one of the best overall exercises there is. Even though you do not have access to a pool or don't know how to swim, you can actually do swimming movements wherever you are. Try this **Swimming Exercise.**

Start with your feet a shoulder width apart and your knees slightly bent. Bend over at the waist and stretch out your right arm as far as possible, keeping it close to your ear as you come up. Do the same with the left arm. Now make crawl swimming motions with your arms. Begin with 20 each side and work up to 100. If you are more advanced, lie face down across an armless chair and do the overhead crawl, flutter kicking your legs at the same time. Start out easy and don't overdo it. The swimming movement helps develop the arms and chest as well as the shoulders. It also aids in strengthening the lower back and leg muscles and is excellent for posture. Breathe in through your nose and exhale through your mouth, contracting your stomach muscles as you breathe out.

Now let's try some more exercises for your chest.

**Chair Push-ups:** Stand with your feet a shoulder width apart, facing the chair; bend at the waist and grasp the sides of the chair seat. Keeping the 45-degree bend in your waist, and bending only at the waist, lower your chin to the seat of the chair. Pause and push yourself back up. Start out by doing as many as you can; don't overdo it and work up to doing 15 at a time.

Another great chest exercise can be done in any part of your house, office, etc. All you need is a bare wall.

**Wall Push-ups:** Stand about two feet from a wall, with your legs a shoulder width apart. Lean forward against the wall and spread your hands a shoulder width apart. Push yourself away from the wall until your arms are straight. Pause and then lower yourself back toward the wall. Again, start out by doing as many as you are able to and work up to doing 20 at a time.

If you have a bench handy, or you can use the end of your bed, try this exercise for your chest.

**Pullovers:** Lie on your back on the edge of a bed or bench. Using a book, iron, or something else that will provide weight, extend the weight (held in both hands) straight up toward the ceiling. Keeping your arms straight, lower the weight down behind your head, pause, and slowly raise the weight until it is once again above your head. Start with a small weight and increase it as you become stronger. Do this movement slowly. Start out doing 4 or 5 and work up to 15 repetitions.

There are rewards in fitness, for example the axiom, "Healthy body, healthy mind." A glowing awakening after

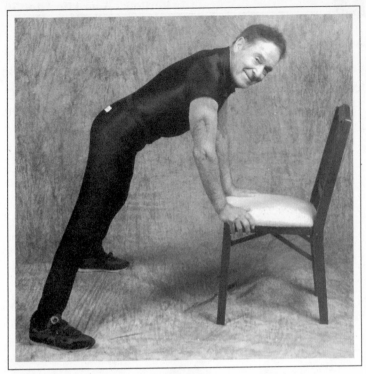

**Chair push-ups: 1st position**

**Chair push-ups: 2nd position**

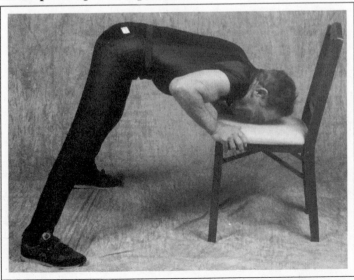

a healthy night's sleep is just one reward you experience every morning. It carries you through the toughest challenges every day and allows you to relax in the evening. These are yours now, in whatever measure you wish, if you will continue along with me.

# Chapter 6

# Chart a Course

I'm sure most of you have read this Proverb in the Bible, "As a man thinketh in his heart so is he." If you adhere to this philosophy then if you think you are over the hill you are over the hill. It's a self-fulfilling prophecy—"I'm too old to change, so why try?"

A lethargy sets in. You have, let's say, the excuse of putting things off until tomorrow; particularly the personal improvement things. But we know tomorrow never comes! So grows the art of procrastination, one of the fatal side effects of fiftysomething.

You may decide, for example, that it would be wise to take off pounds and tighten up the old waistline. You know how to do it of course: counting calories and doing some simple exercises. "Not this minute," says your lazy mind. You decide you'll start tomorrow but you never really get started.

Excuses and procrastination are the major causes of being out of shape. People prepare themselves for failure by putting things off and coming up with reasons not to exercise or follow proper diets. Instead of making up excuses for not exercising and eating properly, list the reasons why you should.

Find something that will remind you to exercise every day. My friends Raechel and Bill Parker have their own unique ways of getting started. Bill does it by putting on his sweats, then he knows he has to exercise. Raechel, who likes to procrastinate, starts to stretch just when she feels the urge to put off exercising until tomorrow. By warming up with the stretches she prepares herself to continue into her exercise routine.

With new inroads in communications, some cable companies will sell you a gadget that opens the windows, turns on the TV, turns the radio on and off, or starts the CD player. The only thing they haven't figured out is how to do your exercises for you.

No wonder life can become a discontented, drifting experience; a trap that can soften you physically and mentally; a ship without a rudder. If this is the case, what we need is a rudder and a schedule to follow.

If you were going to make a long motor trip through new areas, you certainly would check the oil, gasoline, and tire pressure and consult road maps before you started. Then as you go, you'll pay attention to road signs and landmarks to see that you don't stray off course. If we stay on a course and develop new habits, a new outlook, new healthy attitudes toward eating, drinking, and exercising, we will proceed faster and stronger. The route will be gradual but steady. It's like the snail—he doesn't move very fast but he gets the job done. Remember the tortoise and the hare story? Patience and planning won the race.

It's easy to see progress in body dimension no matter how slow. As you progress along your charted course, simply step on the scales and measure your arms, hips, chest, and legs to see your improvement. (Use a measurement chart to record your progress.) But there are other effects to be measured such as blood pressure, heart rate, blood sugar level, stress testing, etc. Once everything is working better your body responds, and so does your mind.

It's also important to check such unpredictable factors as mood, disposition, and attitude even though these are subjective and hard to measure.

I'm going to try to establish some roadsigns and landmarks for your convenience. See the checklist on pages 40–41 to show you where you stand right now. You'll have to do the measuring and weighing yourself. Once you start, it can only get better.

Continue to check and recheck this list, making it a point to bring about some improvement in the areas that you feel need it. By all means, feel free to add or subtract from the list to fit your personal needs. Have your spouse or a family member help you come up with suggestions. The point here is to continue improving yourself so that you too can say, as Elaine's mother used to say, "Every day, in every way, I'm getting better and better."

## Self-Improvement Checklist

| | True | Sometimes True | Not True |
|---|---|---|---|
| I see my dentist regularly | ❑ | ❑ | ❑ |
| I dress and look tidy and clean | ❑ | ❑ | ❑ |
| I exercise my body regularly | ❑ | ❑ | ❑ |
| I clean my teeth with care | ❑ | ❑ | ❑ |
| I walk feeling vibrantly alive | ❑ | ❑ | ❑ |
| I walk tall and carry my shoulders erect | ❑ | ❑ | ❑ |
| I believe I am in good health | ❑ | ❑ | ❑ |
| I don't take sleeping pills or laxatives | ❑ | ❑ | ❑ |
| I can, and will, do 10 half-situps or 10 push-ups right now | ❑ | ❑ | ❑ |
| I want to look healthy and fit | ❑ | ❑ | ❑ |
| Cigarettes aren't necessary for my happiness | ❑ | ❑ | ❑ |
| I pass up dessert if I've eaten enough | ❑ | ❑ | ❑ |
| I am moderate in my alcohol consumption | ❑ | ❑ | ❑ |
| I eat a healthy breakfast every day | ❑ | ❑ | ❑ |
| Meals are a positive part of my day | ❑ | ❑ | ❑ |
| I keep fresh fruit and vegetables handy | ❑ | ❑ | ❑ |
| I complimented my husband/wife today | ❑ | ❑ | ❑ |
| I am pleasant to waitresses, cab drivers, etc. | ❑ | ❑ | ❑ |
| I answer letters promptly | ❑ | ❑ | ❑ |
| I give other drivers the right of way with courtesy | ❑ | ❑ | ❑ |
| I never refuse to dance | ❑ | ❑ | ❑ |

|  | True | Sometimes True | Not True |
|---|:---:|:---:|:---:|
| People are glad to see me arrive | ❏ | ❏ | ❏ |
| I am a cheerful person | ❏ | ❏ | ❏ |
| I am comfortable listening while others converse | ❏ | ❏ | ❏ |
| I am not critical of other people or age groups | ❏ | ❏ | ❏ |
| I try to increase my vocabulary and use new words every week | ❏ | ❏ | ❏ |
| I have read 20 of the world's literary classics | ❏ | ❏ | ❏ |
| I am getting everything possible out of my career | ❏ | ❏ | ❏ |
| I am willing to work hard | ❏ | ❏ | ❏ |
| I meditate on wise words I hear | ❏ | ❏ | ❏ |
| I find it easy to say "I'm sorry" | ❏ | ❏ | ❏ |
| I can say "I don't know" | ❏ | ❏ | ❏ |
| I don't admit defeat easily | ❏ | ❏ | ❏ |
| I don't complain about my age | ❏ | ❏ | ❏ |
| I can accept advice | ❏ | ❏ | ❏ |
| My physical-marital relations are first-rate | ❏ | ❏ | ❏ |
| I believe I have many productive years ahead of me | ❏ | ❏ | ❏ |
| I believe life generally has gone well for me | ❏ | ❏ | ❏ |
| I can be as romantic as I ever was | ❏ | ❏ | ❏ |
| I welcome the start of each new day | ❏ | ❏ | ❏ |
| I go to sleep easily at night and sleep soundly | ❏ | ❏ | ❏ |
| It doesn't embarrass me to be "a little silly" at times | ❏ | ❏ | ❏ |
| I don't make excuses for my shortcomings | ❏ | ❏ | ❏ |

# Chapter 7

# Haste Makes Waste— Have a Plan

Some things in life are self-evident. Drive your car too fast and you get a ticket. Eat too fast and too much you feel bloated. Try to change your daily habits too abruptly and you end up changing nothing. It's human nature.

Keep this in mind as we go along. It's difficult to change overnight but if you are persistent and take one step at a time you will see results.

The key is consistency. Day by day you will change very little, but if you drop something harmful from your life each day and add something beneficial, before long, you'll begin to notice a difference.

Get on a schedule of adding and subtracting, trying not to take on more than you could reasonably handle. Scheduled consistency is what does the job. I find that students always do better when they plan today what they expect to accomplish tomorrow. Today, for instance, you might substitute an apple for a calorie-loaded dessert. Tomorrow you might get off that soft chair and try at least five simple exercises. You'll be that much further along than you are today.

Planning brings order into busy lives. It gives you a mindset, a purpose with direction and it's the first step to getting started. It overcomes inertia, the "couch potato" syndrome. With a plan, like getting out of bed at 7:00 A.M., we are mentally more likely to do it. Follow that plan by doing something each day, no matter how small, and *it will get done*. Without a commitment it's too easy to put it off. It's even easier to miss the second day. Then you're back in the procrastination rut that got you into this condition in the first place.

The late ballet star Rudolf Nureyev once commented on missing his daily conditioning routine. "If I miss a day, I know it. If I miss two days, my fellow dancers know it. If I miss three days, the audience knows it."

Any major deviation in our daily lives produces a reaction. If you suddenly started a strenuous exercise program, you'd be stiff and sore the next day. If you eat less food than normal, you'd soon have hunger pangs. You want to start out gradually and work up to your goal. Making changes later in life can be a fun-filled, fruitful, inspiring experience. Let's not ruin it by overdoing it and getting discouraged too soon.

When I met Elaine, she hadn't exercised in years. I gave her a program to work on, but she became overly enthusiastic and suffered the consequences of becoming stiff and sore. A good example of haste makes waste. The mind might tell you that you are in shape but the body knows otherwise. That's why we must learn to make haste slowly.

Just do a little each day as directed. Enthusiasm must be used skillfully. The improvements will come as part and parcel of new habits we want to form. The more anything becomes habit the less effort it requires and the easier it is. You are the sum total of your habits. It is what makes you what you are and it makes Jack LaLanne what he is. You can improve any facet of your life, whether it be making money, relationships, eating nourishing foods, exercise, changing your hair style, or even the clothes you wear. All it takes is changing a few bad habits for a few good habits.

Right now, let's make one small adjustment in the way you eat. Maybe you're out of shape because of a fondness for candy, cake, ice cream, or pie. These are laden with sugar and empty calories. Calories make fat and fat makes you older than your years. Let's see if we can't wean you off sugar indulgence and suggest something more rejuvenating.

At the time I attended Paul Bragg's health lecture at the age of 15, I was a sugarholic, but had the desire to quit cold turkey, which I did. I realize that not everyone can do that, so we must take each step at a time. Let's simply work some different sweets into your daily diet.

Today it will be enough to eat one piece of fresh fruit instead of ice cream or pie. Try a cookie; there are many cookies on the market sweetened with fruit juice instead of sugar. Try a little grated apple with lemon juice or a mashed banana for desert. Simply mash a banana with a fork until it looks like a pudding, mix in a little lemon juice, and put it in a dessert dish with a fresh strawberry on top and *voilà!*, you have a gourmet dessert.

At this point I have to tell you a little story about Dennis James, whom you probably remember from television. One day after we had played golf he mentioned that he loved desserts. I asked him to leave the room for a few minutes and I would make him a dessert he would love. I mashed a banana the way I just described it to you. He came back into the room, took a spoonful and couldn't believe his taste buds. When I told him it was a mashed banana he was pleasantly surprised, especially when he learned that it had only 80 calories and was high in potassium and phosphorus. That was twenty years ago and he still eats my banana surprise. Try it, you'll like it.

Fruit for dessert at one meal isn't such a radical change in your diet. If you did no more than cut out a major source of excess sugar, you'd avoid thousands of calories while losing weight in the course of a year.

This, in fact, is what a 50-year-old friend of mine did to reduce his weight from 250 to 175 pounds. He slowly changed a few habits. He quit eating between-meal snacks, substituted low-calorie soups instead of creamy soups, cut out cream in his coffee, traded low-calorie dressing for his favorite blue cheese dressing, nonfat milk for whole milk, nonfat frozen yogurt for high-calorie ice cream and egg white omelets for bacon and eggs. These are just a few of the changes he made. It's really easy when you start with just one change at a time.

Now let's attack the matter of fried food. Research shows that most Americans eat more fried food than is good for them and far more than is necessary. Fried foods have added more inches to waistlines than any other single factor (except the lack of exercise). If you want that lean, trim look of vital fitness, let's see if we can make one small change.

Eggs are a wonderful source of nutrients. Health professionals agree that four whole eggs (or yolks) a week are acceptable. An egg can be soft boiled or poached, it doesn't need to be fried. But if you insist that fried or scrambled eggs are an institution with you and you couldn't start the day any other way, lets change a few habits. Instead of butter, use a little canola or olive oil to fry or scramble your eggs. If you are eating breakfast in a restaurant, tell the waitress or waiter you want your eggs scrambled dry or try Egg Beaters℠ (they taste just like eggs) and you'll ingest fewer calories. Personally, I use just the egg whites; scrambled, in omelets or hard boiled. Why? Egg whites have about 15 calories while the whole egg has about 70, and an egg white has 7 grams of protein and no fat. Now let's make a comparison between egg whites and a steak. One pound of steak is about 1,000 calories and has around 25 grams of protein. One egg white has 7 grams of protein and 15 calories, so if you eat 4 egg whites you're getting 28 grams of protein and only 60 calories, 5 egg whites give you 75 calories and 35 grams of protein, and so on. Put this on tomorrow's schedule; we're not trying to get the job done in one day.

Somewhere in that schedule make a notation about milk. Many Americans are heavy milk drinkers and I'm not so sure it's good. With artery-clogging, saturated fats in mind, I keep my own consumption of dairy products to a minimum. Don't leap to a hasty conclusion, though. I'm not going to ask you to cut out all milk, fattening though it is at 170 calories per 8-ounce glass. I'm only going to suggest some changes. Instead of whole milk, think of substituting nonfat or skim milk. It starts out tasting a little thin but in a short time, your taste buds re-adjust. Plus nonfat milk will give you taste plus calcium, phosphorus, and protein but with no animal fats.

Be patient when changing habits, it takes approximately six weeks for your body to adjust. Make substitutions slowly. Remember, HASTE MAKES WASTE!

## Chapter 8

# The Way You Look

Many men and women let themselves go and slowly become unkempt as they face the other side of 50. They see a few gray hairs, a couple of laugh lines, some extra pounds and soon evolve into the falling-apart specimen sometimes associated with senior citizens.

This is the worst possible thing you can do. When you give up mentally, physical deterioration is sure to follow. Fortunately, there are some things you can do about it. Grooming and your appearance are among them.

How many really well-groomed men and women of your age group do you notice in everyday life? Look at yourself.

Let's start with the women. Do your shoes have that fresh-from-the-box sparkle or are they scuffed? Are they just comfortable, or are they comfortable and smart? How about your fingernails? Are your hands dry and chapped? Could you accept an impromptu lunch date, this very moment, without apologizing for your hair?

Go to the beauty shop and get a brand-new hair-do. Have the beautician do your hair in the very youngest style that you can wear. Color it if that will perk you up. You'll smile to yourself when you see it and you'll act as young as you look.

Go with the latest clothing styles. As women grow a little older, they tend to wear the same old things without any consideration for the seasons. If you feel embarrassed when your car is out of date, and keeps breaking down, you yearn for a newer model. Feel the same about your personal appearance. Trade yourself in for a newer model, in this case, the newer you.

You must somehow be so attractive to the man in your life that he cannot become disinterested. Grooming is a great big visual boost to your morale and to his.

It's just as true for men. Sex drive comes from the subconscious. The man who fears that he can't attract the opposite sex very likely telegraphs that feeling through his appearance. Shoes not shined the way they were in his courting days. Shirt laundered but still wrinkled. The billowing bulges at his waistline are hanging over his pants. Is this man saying he is finished?

I urge this man to put something on his schedule right now. Get yourself a styled haircut and a manicure. You've never had one? Try it, you'll get a million-dollar lift. Every time you (or anyone else) looks at those clean, professionally trimmed nails you'll feel good all over. You'll have taken one step down the age ladder. I work out at the gym with great athletes and I get my nails manicured every time I get my hair cut. No one calls me a sissy!

Go to your closet, get those outdated clothes and give them away. Go out this afternoon and buy yourself something new. I mean this literally. Do it right away. You'll want it as a symbol of the changes we're about to make. Don't buy a new suit or dress just yet. Wait a few weeks until you've trimmed down a little so you can buy a smaller size.

Wear clothes that are flattering to your particular body style. Be color coordinated. Just because something is in style doesn't mean it's for you. Accentuate your good features. Good taste never goes out of style.

I consider it wise for a person to go through his or her wardrobe regularly and throw things away. Make room for the new, it's necessary to good grooming. It's like throwing away the months and, with them, some of the years. It has always worked for me and I continue to be a self-confident man in my eighties. I wasn't always self-confident, I assure you. I used to have to do all kinds of things to cheer myself up. One of them was to deliberately buy a new suit just when my better judgment shrieked, "You can't afford it, Jack." I did that many times and learned to scrimp and save on other things. I always felt better for it. It boosted my morale. I felt self-assured when I went out in public. I did a better job of everything I tried.

Being well groomed is not a matter of money. It's a matter of spending a little time, effort, and thought. A man may spend a fortune on his clothes and ruin the whole effect with a sloppy shirt and tie; another man with only $100 to spend on a suit can be impeccably dressed.

As a matter of fact, as we proceed into the later chapters, those designed to improve your body, you'll find that it will save you money. The more you condition your body with my trimnastics and guided nutrition, the easier it is to find bargains in clothes that fit you. Keep in mind, it isn't easy to look well groomed when your belly is bulging. You will be able to try on trousers and jackets that fit—for a change.

Change is part of our program for you. The compliments

you get will make the other changes in the program easier to accomplish. It's important to remember that you're working from the outside in. If you look younger you'll feel younger, and vice versa.

People who do this, I've discovered, seem to follow through better on their diets. They work out better with their exercises. Everything they try goes better. They are more relaxed and start to read better books, find more engrossing hobbies, learn languages, new dances, new manners. They're alive, proud, and competent. They develop confidence, enthusiasm, and a zest for living that defies aging. For them there is no fear of romance's flying out the window, no complaints of sexual impotence.

It may sound egotistical to you—but is it ego to want to look your best? To be admired? To be attractive to the opposite sex? If it makes you feel good, how bad can it be? That's the way life is. Your neighbors must feel the same way. Why else would they bathe? Shave? Get a haircut? Clean their houses, make the beds, or get the car washed? It isn't all ego, it's common sense to care what people think of you. We're not hermits, we live in a society of men and women who would be mighty ugly if they didn't take some pride in caring for themselves.

Grooming, I insist, is vital to our health and vitality after our fifties. It's our first visual aid to satisfaction with ourselves. Won't you do something about yours today?

# Chapter 9

# Add a Little Faith

I believe that having faith is a part of any self-improvement program. There has to be an omnipotent power that puts everything together. Nature shows us this every day of our lives. Having faith reminds me of a little story I often tell in my lectures.

Johnny was a little kid whose goal was to win a race at school. He participated in every race but was always dead last. The final race of the season was in progress and, as usual, Johnny was running last. All of a sudden halfway through the race Johnny started talking to himself and he began to run faster and faster. He passed one, then another and another and pretty soon he was in front and he won the race! His coach said, "I can't believe it Johnny, I can't believe it! I saw you talking to yourself out there, what were you saying?" Johnny answered, "I wasn't talking to myself, I was talking to God." The coach asked, "What were you saying to God?" Johnny replied, "Dear God you lift my legs up and I'll put them down, dear God you lift my legs up and I'll put them down."

We all need a little help from time to time. You cannot be in my profession of physical fitness (connected with the mind and the body) and not believe that there is a supreme being that keeps this universe together. Do you think that humans could make a calculator like our brain or a pumping system like our heart? The heart is an indestructible muscle that goes on ad infinitum; the only way you can hurt it is when the circulation going to the heart is impaired. Do you think that humans could ever devise a filtering system like our kidneys or a laboratory like our liver? Do you think that science could ever make a machine that can be damaged only by a lack of use? Do you think that we could ever create a machine that changes constantly? Each one of the seventy trillion cells in the body changes every sixty to ninety days (except the central nervous system), helping to reverse the aging process. Yes, "We are wonderfully and fearfully made!"

I'm concerned with living the life we have and living it vibrantly and in good health. This, without question, involves the awareness of a creator, no matter how we conceive it. It means spiritual exercises—prayer and meditation—for the development of our inner selves as well as deeper thought on this wonderful life and body we have been given. Our bodies are truly God's living temple but how many of us treat it reverently? Too many of us take it for granted.

The way I see it, two great things in life are feeling well and looking well and two additional things are vitamins F and G. Faith and God. Without them nothing positive is going to happen in our lives. We need faith in something, whether it be faith in God or faith in oneself. So many Americans don't believe in anything, not God, not their country, not themselves. They're like ships without a rudder drifting aimlessly along. Later I'll give you schedules of exercise and nutrition for your physical body. Right now

I want to reemphasize the threefold nature of the LaLanne program.

1. Nourish the body through wise nutrition and exercise.
2. Nourish the mind through intellectual activity, reading, listening, and observing.
3. Nourish the spirit through prayer and meditation.

Why shouldn't prayers be an integral part of a program to build health and vitality? It was the "faith of our forebears" that is credited with building this great nation out of the confusion and conflict of its beginnings. The great and wise Founding Fathers were not reluctant to ask for help and guidance. Neither were the wonderful men and women who pushed on across the continent in covered wagons to fulfill the infant nation's destiny. George Washington often sought divine guidance when the job seemed beyond his mortal powers. Abraham Lincoln, though a communicant of no formal religious congregation, frankly went to his knees when perplexities all but overwhelmed him.

There are as many twists and turns in the process of aging as in the running of a great country or a large corporation.

Recently, in a television interview, a famous director was asked about fear. Particularly, the fear of failure in expensive undertakings. His comment was that, of course he knew fear. He went on to say that most all good actors "suffer" a fear of failure before going on stage. Star athletes feel the same fear before the bell rings or the ball is kicked off. Fear is one crippling factor at work in all of us. As we age, it seems to get easier to fear more things.

I remember how it was in the Great Depression when

men and women lost their jobs. They sat moping and worrying. You could almost see them age. Men of 35 and 40 became old overnight. Their hair seemed to turn gray faster, lines appeared in their faces, their shoulders sagged. They lacked the confidence to seek the few jobs that were open. Franklin D. Roosevelt, a great man who had overcome emotional and physical handicaps himself, reminded the nation, "All we have to fear is fear itself." You can believe that he knew how to use prayer in his life.

There are ways of overcoming fear and other crippling states of mind. You have to find your own way. There are many entrances to your faith and each faith has its own door.

Obviously we will all come to the day when we'll pass on to our next expression of life. While we're here, why not make the most of it?

Banish fear, frustration, and worry. Gain energy by doing. Learn to relax, nap, and find peace of mind.

## Chapter 10

# Into Action

Bend, twist, stretch. That's youth, vitality, movement, and action. Exercise can make you feel young and give you a leg-up on longevity. It can perform miracles on our bodies as well as our personalities.

Let's demonstrate by trying one of my special multipurpose exercises. You'll gain many benefits from this particular one, including a quick insight into how much you may have let yourself slip. I call it my **Get-up and Get-down Exercise.** The purpose of this exercise is to get yourself down on the floor and back on your feet by any means possible. The more awkward you are the better. You'll be making more muscles work. After several tries, the get-ups and get-downs will become a smooth, lithe maneuver showing just how swiftly you can skip back to youth's limber movements.

Remember to get a physical before starting to exercise and seek advice on the pace at which you should start a fitness program.

Get-up and get-downs start easily enough. Simply stand where you are (preferably on a rug) and slowly let yourself down on the floor. Do it any way you can and sprawl out on your back. Now get up again, on your feet, whichever way is easiest. The more overweight you are the more difficult it will be, so be careful. Try the Get-up and Get-down Exercise at least once or twice the first day. If you feel comfortable, try adding another the next day. As your strength and endurance increase, you can add more repetitions. When you become stronger and more flexible, work up to the point where you can do it 15 times or more. This exercise helps your reflexes, coordination, and flexibility along with strengthening your arms, legs, and stomach. To break the monotony, do the exercise as fast as you can then as slowly as you can.

You'll find it's fun getting down on the floor and back on your feet by any means possible. Your whole body's in the act and you're burning calories at the same time.

As you gain in agility, which you will, make a little game of get-up and get-downs. Challenge your mate, children, grandchildren, and friends to try it. Kids really love it. Everyone will have fun doing them and no one can say that you are "over any hill."

Once more, before reading the next paragraph, do a another get-up and get-down.

Breathing a little hard? That's wonderful. Deep breathing isn't a sign you're falling apart, it's one of the healthiest activities you can do. I like the way Dr. A. L. Chapman, former chief of special services for the U.S. Public Health Service, once explained what goes on in your body after exercising and it's no different today. "The blood vessels are lined with smooth muscle fibers. If these smooth muscles don't get enough exercise they atrophy. The only way you can exercise a blood vessel is to create a demand for oxygen in the blood stream." Exercise a blood vessel? Read on! "When you exercise, your muscular tissues use oxygen. Your heart has to beat faster to pump a new supply of oxygen-carrying blood to meet the demand. As your heart increases its pumping action it pushes more blood through the system. The blood vessels expand to allow this more profuse circulation, and then it contracts. This expansion and contraction is exercise."

In other words, your arteries are similar to a water hose. If you push water through it with high force, sedimentation does not accumulate on the wall of the hose. As you exercise you dilate the blood vessels. They expand and contract. This expansion and contraction moves along the sedimentation in your blood vessels, bringing oxygen to all parts of your body and helping to prevent heart problems.

Life itself is in your breath. You might do without food for a week, without water for at least a day, but how long can you go without a breath? (A minute?)

Obviously, we need air when we're sitting, but we need it more, the faster our heart beats, in order to pump along new oxygen supplies. It is estimated that only one-half of one percent of us fill our lungs to capacity as we should.

I want you to learn "body breathing" as the trainers of athletes teach it. We want to get your whole upper body into your breathing. Here's how it's done. Breathe in slowly, through your nose, as though there were a great big balloon inside you to be inflated. Keep inhaling, feel the air filling the diaphragm and the abdomen. You're full to bursting? Exhale hard through your open mouth. Try it again. Purse your lips and start that slow inhaling through your nose. Fill your lungs, feel the lower abdomen tighten as it fills. Stand tall (think of good posture), fling your arms wide, open your mouth, and spill out the air.

Practice this breathing as often as you find time. Try it

when you're tense and tired. Do it at night before going to bed and feel the tension ooze out of you.

Let's try a little exercise to loosen up your spine and really break down that stiffness. I call it my **Bend Over Stretch**. Stand with your legs a shoulder width apart, knees slightly bent. Bend forward and grasp your legs just below and behind the knee. Bring your head forward as if to touch it to the floor. Then come to an erect position again and with your hands on hips, knees slightly bent, bend backward on your braced feet, stretching back as far as you can, trying to look at the wall behind you. Feel the kinks coming out? Go through the exercise slowly several times, advancing the tempo as you gain confidence and coordination. After completing the exercise, inhale deeply, as you just learned to do, and blow out the breath though your mouth.

Some may wonder why this fitness explosion in America? Why are we so different from our parents and our grandparents? Didn't they live to a ripe old age without all this effort? Some did and some didn't.

The answer is simple: Our parents and especially our grandparents had to do more physical labor. Today, with modern science and technology, our lives are filled with labor-saving machines, gadgets, and devices that do miraculous things for and to us.

Several decades ago Dr. Edgar A. Gordon analyzed just what one of these machines does. He noted that "a stenographer, 63 inches tall and weighing 120 pounds, operating a mechanical typewriter uses 87.7 calories per hour. She changed to an electric typewriter and her energy requirement fell to 72.9 calories per hour. Thus there is a saving of 14.8 calories, which for a six-hour day amounts to 90 calories and in a five-day week, to 450 calories. If her food intake and physical activity otherwise remain unchanged, she will gain one pound of body weight in ten weeks because she changed to an electric typewriter." Wow! And now computers let her expend even fewer calories.

Here are some more exercises to help burn off more of those calories.

The first exercise is a tension reliever and can be done anywhere, even right by your desk. These **Shoulder Shrugs** can be done sitting in a chair or standing. Allow your shoulders to shrug. Bring your shoulders up toward your ears (if you can touch your ears you have long ears), push your shoulders back trying to touch your shoulder blades together, then return to a relaxed position. Begin with 10 repetitions. Do them several times a day to relieve nervous tension and to bring blood to the upper body.

As we age, many of us complain of flabby upper arms.

**Shoulder shrugs**

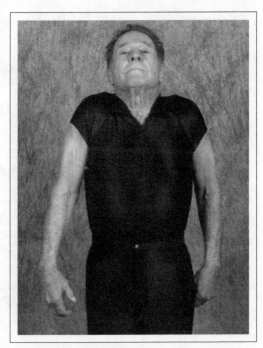

Try these **Biceps Curls.** Stand tall, waist in, with arms down to sides, palms facing forward. Clench your fists and bring them up to your shoulders, pretending your elbows are glued to your sides. These are great for the front of the arms. Do them 10 or 15 times. As you advance you can use books or dumbbells.

**Biceps curls: 1st position**     **Biceps curls: 2nd position**

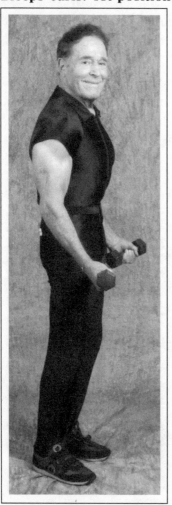
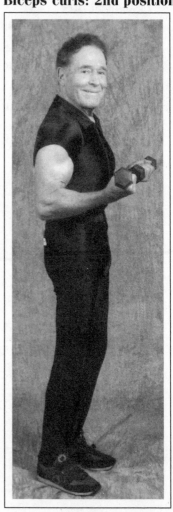

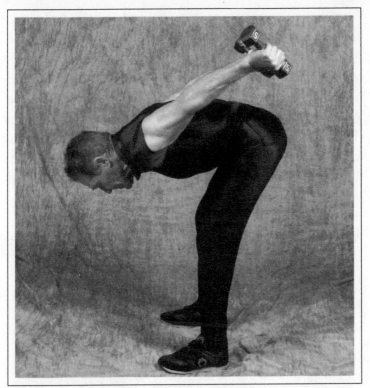

**Triceps extensions**

Here's one for the back of the arms, **Triceps Extensions**. Stand with your legs a shoulder width apart. Bend over at the waist, keeping your elbows close to your side and as high as possible. Then extend arms to the back with a smooth extension movement, trying to touch the ceiling. This helps strengthen the muscles in the back of the arms. If you need more resistance you can use extra weights.

While you're in this position here's one for the upper back, **Bent Over Rows**. Bend over at the waist so that your torso is parallel to the floor. Knees bent. Let your arms hang to the floor. Clench your fists and raise your elbows toward the ceiling, keeping them as close to your body as possible.

Dumbbells or books can also be used for greater muscle challenge.

Now let's get your blood pumping to burn calories. This one is called the **Windmill**. Bend over at the waist, contracting your abdominal muscles, keeping knees slightly bent. With your arms stretched out, simultaneously swing your right arm across your body and try to touch your left hand to the ceiling. Then swing back your left arm and extend the right hand to the ceiling. Do this one as rapidly as possible.

**Windmill**

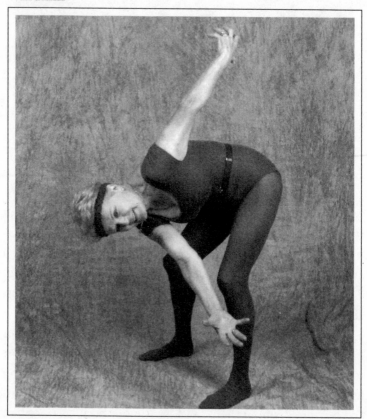

I'm often asked the question, "How long and what time of day should I work out?" Working out is a very personal matter. It depends on whether you're going out for serious body building or keeping your body in condition. For the average person I suggest that they work out at least 20 to 30 minutes and change their program every 2 to 3 weeks. Some people like to work out in the morning and then again in the evening. However much time you need, or wish to give, will be up to you. The payoff depends on what you invest.

I recently read an interview with a 68-year-old New York City executive who was kidnapped and held prisoner in a dark cave for nearly two weeks. He came out of his harrowing ordeal in excellent shape, though he received little food and water. How? He kept his mind and body active. As a Marine Corps lieutenant he had seen combat in World War II. After the war he exercised and stayed in excellent physical shape. Though he lost 18 pounds during his imprisonment, he returned to work within a few days and credits his Marine training for his survival. Had he not been in good shape he may not have survived.

What I want you to get from life is inner peace, tranquillity, release of nervous tensions, and fitness for the years you're living. I want you to have that alive, vibrant, good feeling that goes with health plus fitness.

"Probably one of the best ways to counteract the harmful effect of nervous tension," said the famous cardiologist Dr. Paul Dudley White, "is physical fatigue from healthy exercise."

Too many people have forgotten or never knew this. They sit themselves into bad health. Dr. William Rabb coined the term "loafer's heart" (the reverse of athlete's heart) and reported with his international team of medical researchers that prolonged physical inactivity causes an outpouring of adrenalinelike hormones that produce degenerative changes in the heart muscle and chambers.

One of his other studies diagnosed another disease or deficiency, which he called "television leg." It is a weakness of the lower extremities that interferes with the ability to run and walk properly and is a result of excessive sitting in front of the TV. The newest name for that is "couch potato." Dr. Rabb also noted that in older people, blood clots are becoming increasingly common, a result of prolonged television sitting, which hampers circulation.

I suspect a lot of us, who aren't generally guilty of this, can still get the general idea from what happens to us every year at World Series or Super Bowl time. Let me suggest a little precautionary exercise for a prolonged television sitter. Get off that soft seat every half hour. Breathing deeply, stand up on your tip toes and reach for the ceiling, try to touch the ceiling (if you do, you are very tall) and hold for a count of 5. Now with your knees slightly bent (bending your knees helps take the strain off your back), bend over at the waist and try to touch your palms on the floor. Maybe you can only touch your knee or your ankle the first day, then try to go a little farther each day without straining yourself. Keep in mind, the body responds only when it is challenged beyond what it is used to doing. This is a start in helping to reverse the aging process. You'll limber up your whole body, get the blood flowing, and make watching the game more enjoyable. You'll also be doing something to counteract numbness, the couch potato syndrome, television leg, and loafer's heart.

Dr. White was way ahead of his time when he said, "I believe that the physiological effect of regular exercise throughout one's life will probably, in time, be proven to be one of the best antidotes against the epidemic development of coronary thrombosis and high blood pressure in this country. Along with exercise, of course, there should be recognition of the wisdom of preventing obesity and of avoiding food heavy with animal fat."

Are you getting the picture? Or maybe you already have.

There are many influences and pressures on us today because we're living in a tense and troubled world. Though we've seen the end of communism in the Soviet Union there are still twenty-two separate wars going on around the globe. As we used to say when I was in the South Pacific during World War II, "We're sweating it out." Well, let's literally sweat it out, with exercise. Perspiring is good for us. It's nature's way of cleansing our bodies from the inside out. It gets rid of all our impurities and it's excellent for our skin.

There's another way to live in a tense world. I feel it is very important to recharge your battery. Learn to take naps. Even if you can seize five to ten minutes, take a little catnap. Many successful businessmen do and more should. When you awaken splash your face with cold water, take half a dozen deep breaths and you'll be surprised how clear your mind functions. What do babies and animals do after they eat? Sleep! People in Latin and European countries take two- to three-hour lunches. We here in America go at such a fast pace we don't have time for naps and end up tense and tired.

Getting into action means you're becoming a positive doer. So far I've offered several good exercises for you to try. Make a little schedule for yourself and plan a time for these exercises.

In the next chapter I'll be offering you a series of **Magic Fives** exercises for everyday use. I call them my Magic Fives because I feel the results will be like magic.

# Chapter 11

# My Magic Fives

Now for my **Magic Fives**—five simple exercises you can do in your own home or office with only a straight chair and two books as your "gym equipment." Working out with professionally made, resistive, gym equipment is always preferable but these exercises can be done in between your regular workouts

Let's say that you are not overweight or underweight and that you just need a set of quick-to-do exercises that will gently tighten and firm your body to its youthful look.

These five will help you do the job if you're really diligent. Do the same five exercises four or five times a week. That's the real magic for you Fifties-or-over. All other exercises in this book will revolve around the Magic Fives.

These five will reach to almost every part of your body, from the soles of your feet to the top of your head. You may find yourself a little awkward in the beginning but don't worry, coordination will come.

First, go through them slowly from a count of 1 to 10 and feel how they flex a small muscle here, a large one there.

Try each one individually but practice so that you can increase each one and repeat it 10 times before going on to the next. Consider each exercise as a set of 10 repetitions and you'll soon be trained to do all 5 as sets.

I'm asked quite often, what is the difference between a set and a repetition? Okay, let's say that you are doing an exercise and you can do it only 3 times, that's 3 repetitions or 1 set. If you repeat your 3 repetitions 3 times then you have done 3 sets. For instance, if you do an exercise 10 times and you repeat the 10 times again 15 to 30 seconds later you have done 2 sets.

As I describe them I will show you how each exercise benefits which part of your body and how. Return to this section of the book as often as necessary to refresh your memory. Work the Magic Fives every day and revitalize your life.

Let me suggest you work out in front of a mirror. Picture in your mind's eye what you eventually want to look like. As you do your exercises, this visualization will help give you the motivation to reach your goal and help you concentrate more. You can also see if you are doing the exercise correctly. Now for my **Magic Fives:**.

## Swings

The first of my Magic Fives is the Swing Exercise. This is one of my favorite exercises because it works more muscles simultaneously than practically any other one you can do. It is also a good warm-up exercise.

Place a light book between your hands, spread your feet a shoulder width apart, making sure your knees are flexed. Now bend over at the waist and slowly swing the book down between your legs trying to touch the wall behind you, exhaling as you bend. Then still holding the book between your hands, keeping your arms straight, come up to an erect position and try to touch the wall behind you, inhaling as you come up. In other words, as you go down you breathe out and as you come up you breathe in. Do not use jerky movements, but make them slow and smooth. Beginners start out with two or three swings and as you feel more comfortable with the exercise, increase the repetitions. Work up to ten repetitions as a set. Remember everyone is different so you have to go at your own pace. Don't overdo it and don't forget to bend your knees while exercising.

# Knees to Chest

This exercise is excellent for the upper and lower waistline as well as for the hip flexors. It helps strengthen your abdominal muscles and stretches the lower back. Sit in a chair and scoot down so that you are sitting on the edge of the seat almost on your tailbone, while keeping your shoulders against the back of the chair. Grasp the sides of the chair with both hands to maintain your balance. Now draw both knees into your chest (if you can touch your knees to your chest, you've got long knees). If you are unable to lift both knees into your chest, try lifting one knee then the other and work up to using both knees. When you become really advanced, you can try holding a book between your knees as you bring them up to your chest. This exercise can also be done lying on your back on the floor or on the bed. Start out with 2 or 3 and work up to 10 or 15. I can't say this too many times: Make haste slowly. After the Knees to Chest

Exercise keep your same position in the chair and pretend that you are pumping a bicycle. Start with a little bicycle and make little short movements. As you progress you can pretend you are riding an immense bicycle. Now make great big movements by bringing your knee into your chest as far as you can and then extending your leg out as far as it will go, bringing it down close to the floor and back up again. Keep breathing rhythmically the entire time, breathing in through your nose and out through your mouth. Now, as you progress and as you get in better condition, do this very fast, as though somebody were chasing you and you are trying to get away from them. This is a tremendous exercise for your thighs, your waist, and your hip flexors, but it especially burns up a tremendous amount of calories and is a great cardiovascular conditioner. It also helps your reflexes and coordination—and it is fun.

## Leg Lunges

Now here is a great exercise to help you get rid of those flabby, sagging hips. It's also great for your quadriceps (the muscles in front of the thigh that extend the lower leg) and a great strength and endurance builder. Hang on to a chair. Stand to the side, and hang on to the back of it, keeping the body erect. Step forward with your right leg and lunge forward as you have seen swordsmen do in the movies, then come back to the original position and repeat with your left leg. Keep alternating from your right leg to your left and as you get progressively stronger bend the knee more and make a bigger step. Never lean forward during this exercise, always keep erect. I would start out with 2 or 3 on each leg and increase as your condition improves.

# Leg Extensions to the Back

This is tremendous for the back of your legs, lower back, and the back of your neck. In fact, it works all the muscles in the back, from the head all the way down to the bottom of your feet. It is especially effective in firming up the buttocks. Put your hands on the seat of a chair. Bend over at the waist and back away until you are comfortable, keeping your arms straight. Now, lift your right leg as high as possible, pointing your toes. As your leg comes up your head also comes up, as if you were looking at the ceiling. The opposite leg, the one you're standing on, can be bent slightly. When the leg goes down put your chin on your chest and round your back, tensing your abdominal mus-

**Leg extensions**

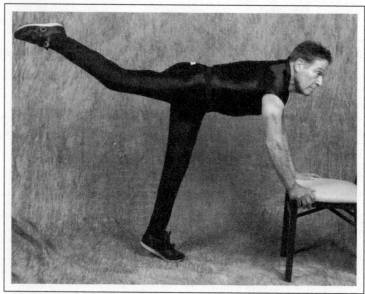

cles. Inhale as the leg comes up, exhale as the leg goes down. Alternate the right leg with the left. Do this exercise very slowly; lift, don't kick and don't jerk. When you are lifting your leg, tense your hips as tightly as possible, and as you lower the leg and you round your back with chin on chest, tense your abdominal muscles. In other words you're working your abdominal muscles when your leg comes down and your hips as the leg comes up.

## Two-Way Punches

Punches work almost every muscle in your upper body and are a great cardiovascular exercise. If you really want to burn up the calories and help trim your waistline, try these.

**Two-way punches**

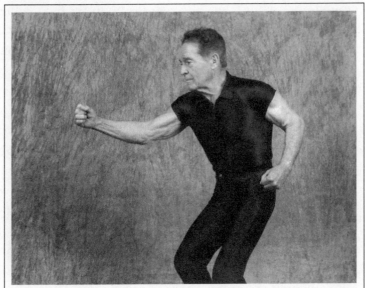

**Forward Punches:** Stand with your feet a shoulder width apart, flex your knees a little bit, stand erect and pretend that you have a punching bag in front of you (just as you've seen boxers working out on a punching bag). Punch it with your right hand as hard as you can, then your left hand, alternating right, left, right, left. Pretend you are punching an invisible bag out there in front of you. Start slowly and increase the pace so that you are punching rather rapidly. As your elbow comes back, try to hit the wall behind you, then as your arm goes forward, try to hit the wall in front of you. In other words, make big, complete movements. I also want you to get a lot of body into this; that's why I want you to bend your knees slightly. Forward punching is helpful not only for the cardiovascular system but also for your arms, shoulders, upper back, and chest.

**Overhead Punches:** Clench your fists, stand erect and punch with your right arm overhead, trying to hit the ceiling, then with your left hand trying to hit the ceiling, dropping your elbow down as low as you can. Do this rapidly. This works the back of your arms, the sides of your waist, and the calves as you go up on your toes. It is very beneficial for your posture and flabby arms.

After you have done the overhead punches, come back to the original position where you were punching forward, only this time pull your waist in and punch with both hands together rapidly trying to hit the wall behind you with your elbows and hit your fists on the wall in front of you. Now immediately punch overhead trying to touch the ceiling with both your fists. As you come down bring your elbows down as low as you can and punch up and down with rapid movements. The faster you punch the more calories you burn. When you become more advanced you can use two books for extra resistance. Remember to breathe deeply, inhaling through your nose and exhaling through you mouth. The more oxygen you get into your bloodstream, the more fat you burn up. After all, you are a combustion engine. It is just like blowing on a fire—the more wind, the faster the fire burns. It's the same way with the human body. That's why I want you to do these exercises vigorously when you get in shape.

# Chapter 12

# Let's Face It

Your face is an open book for all to read. How does your face read? When you look in the mirror, what do you see? A vibrant energetic person in good shape or a tired worn-out soul who has literally given up to the what's-the-use story of neglect. Wrinkles, double chin, rough dry skin, droopy shoulders, or maybe a perpetual pout. Do you see laugh lines or frown lines, good humor or bad humor, joy or unhappiness? These are all telltale signs, written right there on your face. That is just how some people judge the character of others.

Sags and bulges tell plainly of self-indulgence for many men and women as they get older. He likes his food and drink but he's too lazy to exercise. He's sort of a Sloppy Joe. She can't keep her hands out of the chocolate box and she's let herself go. She's gotten careless.

The face is the seat of our expressions and the mirror of our emotions. Bad nutrition, lack of sleep, and worry show in our faces. How we look and feel is a dead giveaway, but only if we let it be.

The texture of the skin is often what broadcasts the fact that we've passed our forty-ninth birthday. The skin is the protective tissue over the facial muscle structure to shelter deeper tissue from injury, drying, and invasion of foreign organisms. It also acts as a thermostat in regulating body temperature. Exercise promotes perspiration, not only in our face, but in the whole body as well. The best of face cleansers help clean the skin, but they can penetrate only so deep. Perspiration cleanses from the inside out.

I have found that people who exercise regularly tend to have younger-looking faces because they are getting blood into the upper extremities. You have over fifty muscles in your face and neck. They help provide a foundation for your facial attractiveness. They are no different than any other muscle in your body—they need to be worked. You can have the world's greatest skin but if the supporting muscles are weak and flabby, you will look years older. Never forget, you are constantly fighting gravity. The face and neck muscles support the skin. When these muscles are exercised it helps firm, tighten, and strengthen them.

The first step to a better-looking face is to try a **Smile** on those facial muscles. Force them a little. Decide that they are going to grow into expressions of character you want the world to see. A smile is a great exercise as it works on both body and spirit. We **Make Faces;** funny faces, contorted faces, grim faces, wry faces, and sad faces. If, for instance, the daily setting of your jaws has caused downbending, stern lines at your mouth, practice upturn smiles forcefully to neutralize the creases. **Smile, grin, show your teeth**. Force the muscle structure around your mouth to pull upward and drag those grim lines out. Now **make all kinds of faces,** open your mouth wide and then purse your lips. Make those muscles move. It takes time, but do a little each day. Remember, it's more difficult to frown than smile.

Perhaps you want to come out from behind that turkey neck, sagging jowls, and double chin that conceal the clean-cut jawline of your younger years. Some of that flab will have to come off by eating properly and cutting down on calories. This includes eating more fresh fruits, vegetables, fish, chicken, and turkey. Now let's go after the neck and chin with an exercise.

**Chin on Chest, Side to Side:** Lie down on a firm surface or sit in a chair with your chin tipped forward toward your chest. Tense your neck muscles and press your chin to your chest. Slowly turn your chin to the left trying to touch your left shoulder. Then turn your head to the right and try to touch your right shoulder. Do this slowly, always keeping your chin on your chest and your neck muscles contracted and tense. Inhale deeply as your head turns. Exhale as you reach the end of the turn. Start with half a dozen turns to the left and to the right and gradually work up to 20, three or four times a week.

This exercise will help rid you of that double chin and firm up your neckline to look more youthful. While you're doing this you're going to help your hair and your eyes. It also helps relieve nervous tension because you are bringing blood to your upper extremities.

**Head Raises:** Lie down across a chair, bed, or bench, face up, and let your head hang over the edge. Lift your head up slowly, do not jerk, and try to touch your chin to your chest, tensing your neck muscles as you come up. Lower your head back down and repeat the exercise 3 or 4 times. As you become more advanced, gently put pressure on your forehead, with your fingertips, as you come up and down. Your fingers act as weight, giving you more resistance. The more resistance given to a muscle the more the muscle is challenged, therefore it responds more readily.

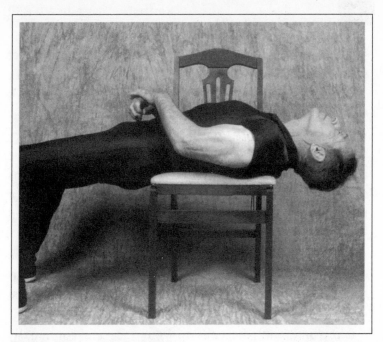

**Head raises: 1st position**

**Head raises: 2nd position**

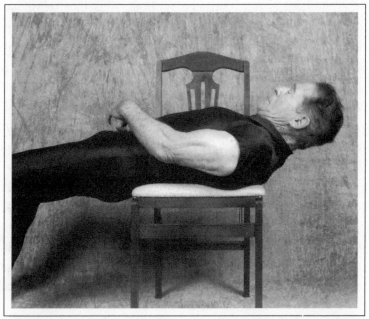

If we overexpose the cells in our face to hours of direct sunlight, they lose many properties that make them work efficiently. Nutrients do not move through the cells as well. Consequently, they become stiff and undernourished, literally forcing age and often causing permanent damage.

I'm sure many of you have friends or relatives who have actually baked in the sun for hours and now their skin has that wrinkled, leathery look. This can also hold true for those who have overexposed themselves to "artificial sun."

If you plan to spend much time in the sun, be sure you coat the exposed areas of your body with a good commercial sun block. Also make sure your head is covered so that your face is shaded.

Keep in mind, the cells in your face are continually dying and new cells are replacing them. Therefore, if you eat more fresh fruits and vegetables and exercise regularly your skin will take on a more youthful glow.

Your face is not complete without your hair. Hair has several functions. It protects the skull from the elements, helps eliminate body wastes from the blood by evaporation through its shafts, and cushions the head from blows. It adds to physical beauty and is also considered an object of adornment. However, our hair has beauty only when it looks healthy, and it looks healthy only when the rest of our body is healthy. When our health generally is down, the hair shows a lack of luster and sheen.

When nutrition is deficient, Mother Nature has a way of conveying this to us. Our hair is one of the first to fade when the normal functions of our body are disturbed. I'm sure you have heard of men and women graying overnight, or hair falling out by the handful. This is definitely a time to see your doctor, but I'm writing this book for those of you who are not ill. If you have surrendered to neglect, I'm here to help you escape. Give your body the raw materials and watch them reflected in your face and hair.

The shafts and root bed of your hair must be kept clean by regular shampooing, otherwise dust and dirt mixed with perspiration and the oil from the sebaceous glands form a crust over the scalp. When this happens new hair can't push through, so give your scalp a good massage while shampooing.

**Scalp Massage:** The best hair exercise is to stand on your head, if you can do it. However, here's one everyone can do. Sit in a chair. Bend over at the waist, head toward floor, between your legs, and let your hands hang down (rag-doll style) to get the blood flowing to the scalp. Massage your scalp, then gently pull your hair all over your head. While in this bent-over position pat your face gently, which brings blood to the face. Another way to get blood flowing to the scalp is to brush and comb your hair frequently.

Exchange grim expressions for smiles and think happier things about this life we're sharing. Being over 50 is not bad at all. It's not much different from 30, really, except we're more mature mentally and most of us a lot more secure materially.

Think about it. Reflect upon it. Let that face of yours show it.

## Chapter 13

# Posture Is the Key

Nothing reveals middle age like posture. It can make you look older or it can make you look younger. Posture reveals as much about you as your face does. If you don't believe me, stand in front of a full-length mirror and slouch, let your shoulders droop. What happens? Your chin drops toward your chest, your stomach pouches out, your breathing becomes shallow, your chest and even your face sag. You become a walking billboard of insecurity and old age. If this is how you go around most of the time, this is how others will see you.

Posture has a lot to do with how one feels about oneself. If you are slumping it prevents good circulation, promotes shallow breathing, and the muscles that support your spine get weak. Whether we are sitting or standing we are always fighting gravity, everything tends to fall from the head to the toes. Many of the 640 muscles in the body are our supporting muscles, and if these muscles are neglected from lack of exercise they lose their supporting ability. When you are fighting gravity, your face, shoulders, chest, and stomach want to droop. This is how many people develop what is known as the "dowager's hump." Bad posture can make you look years older and can help to diminish your energy and vitality; often even your clothes don't fit properly.

A middle-aged woman.

Does your mind's eye complete the picture before I write a single word of description? You don't have to know the color of her hair or eyes. You already have a mental image of a middle-aged woman.

Perhaps a little matronly. A little saggy here and there and trying to hide it under loose clothing.

A middle-aged man.

The same story. He comes out of a catch-all group of people in your mind. Trudging and bulging, stooped shoulders, preoccupied with the cares of middle years. His youth has wandered off. You sense an attitude, an outlook, a posture.

Now let me mention some names: Diana Ross, Joan Collins, Angela Lansbury, Ricardo Mantalban, Debbie Reynolds, Chita Rivera, Clint Eastwood, Lauren Bacall, Jane Fonda, Harry Belafonte, Tina Turner, Sally Kirkland, and Arnold Schwarzenegger.

Here are men and women of 50 or over. So when I said "middle-aged woman" and "middle-aged man," how come your mind's eye didn't select them? I'll tell you why. They don't telegraph their age to most of us. They don't have the posture of neglect.

Let's remember that attraction is the greatest factor in love. No man reacts easily to an unattractive woman and vice versa. Posture is often the key ingredient to attractiveness. A man whose body sags or who has an ungainly potbelly or whose shoulders sag is likely to look too beat most of the time to interest even his loving wife. Similarly, a man may find it impossible to respond amorously to a wife who bulges out of her clothes or is always looking unkempt. The key here is *sex appeal.*

That's the point I'm trying to make as we talk of our posture and what you reveal by it. Posture is one thing we all can improve.

Think of your own group of friends and those few who manage to defy birthdays. Isn't there something special about the set of their heads and their shoulders? Doesn't there seem to be a litheness and elasticity about them that bends with life's buffeting—no stiff, stooped defeat. They seem to command respect and admiration and ooze with confidence.

Nothing reveals middle age like posture. Nothing defies the years like posture. It may add years to your actual age or it may shrug them off. Now, are you ready to throw away the mental crutches and step out with vitality? Or, would you rather stoop under your burdens, bending inevitably toward the grave? Your posture will tell.

Not long ago I received a letter from a creative designer who lives in New York City. "I am one of your faithful students," she said, "and with your continued help I am determined to roll back as many years as I can. I am 52 years of age but I feel 21. All I have to do to prove it to myself is walk out of my apartment building."

She goes on to say that she lives in a building with 1,015 tenants. One-third of them are older men and women who, she protests, should be doing something about their posture. "They're falling apart from disuse and are making themselves look older than they are," the designer reports.

This matter of posture is vital, indeed. It isn't just the sadness of overweight, spreading hips, drooping shoulders, dowager humps, and protruding bellies; there are possible health problems here that poor posture complicates.

Bad posture over a prolonged period can cause the internal organs to be cramped. It is often blamed for much of the trouble women have with their reproductive organs, and can also be a cause of faulty elimination in later years. Also, the heart and lungs are shifted into cramped positions resulting in poor circulation and they can't get the oxygen necessary for their vital functions. Poor posture can also lead to lower-back problems.

Does this offer food for thought to the man or woman who is frustrated by waning sexual powers? It's hard to believe that one can have a satisfactory sex life when he or she is feeling tired and tense.

Right here let's define good posture. Generally the feet in the standing position should point straight ahead. The knees should be flexed just enough to prevent rigidity. The neck is held as straight as possible without losing its normal cervical curve. The chin should be level and nothing must appear forced or tensed about the head position. Shoulders should be down back and relaxed. Hands should hang naturally at the sides, fingers relaxed. When all of this happens the eyes sparkle.

I understand that normal posture varies from man to man or from woman to woman, but did you ever watch a group of proud young Marines marching? The way they carry their bodies, the set of their shoulders, there's no question about posture. However, all of us are not ex-servicemen or women who have had posture training. We should understand that by "civilian posture" we mean that which best suits the individual in accordance with his or her physical condition and environment.

We associate a completely relaxed or slouched posture with laziness. A stately posture, by the same token, seems to say to us that that man or woman has energy, vitality, get-up-and-go.

We aspire to good posture, which we admire, but daily habit is like a daily drug pulling us down. A potbelly, even a small one, is going to pull the head forward and down. The head is, of course, the key to good posture. As the head goes so goes the body. The shoulders will follow the head into this general slump. The arms will sag. Our steps will drag. And so it goes, on and on, from youth into the thirties, the forties, and on through all the years afterward. Get that head up and the body will surely follow.

Good posture begins with the way you walk: head up, arms extended, chest out so you can breathe deeply. Your new posture will show off your physique to its very best advantage. I know a man in his fifties who decided he was weary of losing out romantically—against men his own age. He went into training to lose excess weight, which corrected his posture immediately. Then he threw away his portly wardrobe and bought one to fit his new physique. He was determined to maintain that physique and be guided only by the way his clothes fit. He did very well too, both physically and romantically.

How can we improve our posture at this late date? I have three suggestions. One, quit overeating. Two, start exercising like a young man or woman if you wish to look like one. I can think of no better exercise than my Magic Fives, which I explained in Chapter 11. Start doing them regularly and consistently, but make haste slowly. And three, don't fall back into old habits.

Throw away all of your mental crutches. Help your body to build Mother Nature's girdle. Get limber and loose. Turn to the kind of nutrition that will make you feel buoyant and alive. And strive for a sense of well-being.

Here's a great posture exercise:

**Tiger Stretch:** Stand with your hands clasped loosely behind your back and your feet a shoulder width apart. Extend the clasped hands to arm's length behind you. Now try to touch your shoulder blades together and attempt to reach the wall. While doing this, elevate your head so that you are looking at the ceiling. Feel your shoulders, stomach, and hip muscles tighten? Now bend over at the waist, with knees bent, and look between your legs, hands still clasped at arm's length.

**Tiger stretch**

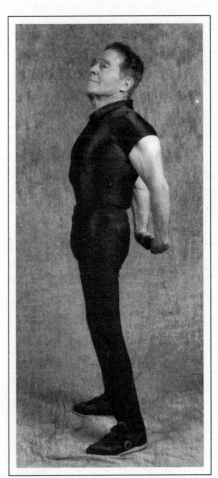

A few more tips to help you improve your posture:

**The Walnut Crack:** Stand tall and pretend you have a walnut between your shoulder blades and a walnut between your buttocks. On the count of 3, crack the imaginary walnuts. Notice what happens to your stomach—it automatically pulls in, instead of pouching out.

**Stomach to Backbone:** Stand tall and let the air out of your lungs. Now attempt to pull your stomach muscles to your backbone. Inhale, and repeat two or three times.

**Pull stomach muscles into backbone**

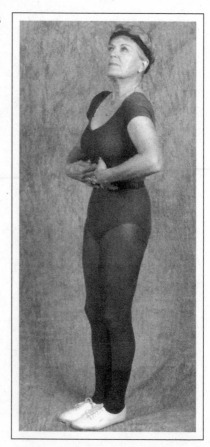

**Waist Away from Belt:** Sitting or standing, pretend you have a tight belt around your waist and attempt to pull your waist away from your tight belt.

**Door-Frame Stretch:** Place your hands on the outside of a door frame approximately shoulder height, fingertips pointing upward. Now attempt to walk through the door and you will find that your hands will hold your shoulders back, giving you a great posture stretch. Try doing this every time you go through a door.

Remember, the world is your mirror and everyone looks at your reflection. Be aware of your posture at all times whether you are sitting or standing. Sit tall! Stand tall!

**Door-frame stretch**

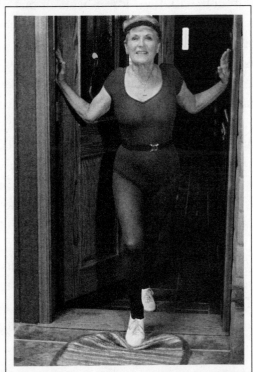

# Chapter 14

# Oh, My Aching Back!

"Oh, my aching back!" How often have you heard this expression? Maybe you have used it many times yourself. There are millions and millions of men and women, young and old, who have trouble with their lower back. In fact in 1992 more people were off work as a result of back problems than any other injury.

The back consists of a bony column supported by muscles. It has three natural curves to help absorb daily stresses and sudden traumas. The center of each curve is where we often feel the ache. These areas are called "cervical" (your neck area), "thoracic" (your midback, behind your chest), and the curve in your low back is called the "lumbar" region. Do you recall the old term "lumbago"? Bear in mind, we are always fighting gravity. When we do not exercise enough, or in the correct way, our muscles cannot perform their supporting function.

Small traumas of life, improper diet, and poor posture can all cause muscle spasm, weakness, and imbalance in muscle strength. This imbalance in supporting strength is the cause of "misaligned" vertebrae and can lead to "pinched nerves," "slipped discs," and "sciatica," among others.

I'll never forget when I first went into business, I was lifting an extremely heavy weight without warming up and pulled a muscle in the left side of my lower back. The muscle went into spasm, which threw my back out of alignment.

Because I knew my myology (the study of the muscles) and kinesiology (the study of movement at the joints), I was able to devise exercises to strengthen the weak side of my back to make it equal to the strong side. If the muscles aren't balanced the stronger muscle takes over and pulls the spine out of alignment, causing discomfort. Your back can go forward, backward, laterally, and around and around, but if it is not in alignment you will not be able to perform these functions efficiently. The muscles that help support and keep your lower back in alignment are:

1. The psoas muscle (the muscle in front of the lumbar spine that connects with the upper thigh bone and bends or raises your leg at the hip)
2. The gluteus maximus (the big muscles in your buttocks)
3. The sacro spinal mass, or the spinus erecti (muscles in the lumbar region that support either side of the spine)
4. The erectus abdominus (the abdominal or stomach muscles)
5. The obliques (the muscles in the sides of the waist that make you bend from side to side)

Later in this chapter I'm going to give you exercises to help strengthen these muscles.

I read recently that at least 80 percent of Americans, many of them over 50, will eventually have a back ailment. The greatest debilitator of backs is neglect. For the most part, individuals who suffer from back problems aren't active enough to keep their muscles and spine limber. A man turns a spadeful of earth and snap! A woman twists to reach a high shelf and ouch! Instead of getting help from a trained expert, they put off seeing a health care professional and perhaps wait weeks and sometimes months for their problem to go away, only to find out that by waiting, the problem has become worse and sometimes chronic. To quote my daughter, Dr. Yvonne LaLanne, who is a chiropractor, "Remember, that pain is the last symptom to appear. By the time we have pain, the misalignment has been long and well established. And even if the pain goes away by itself the misalignment or imbalance is still there waiting for another slight force to push it into our conscious mind."

The best prevention I know for back trouble is fitness. Individuals who keep their bodies firm and limber, who regularly do simple exercises and know about bending the knees when lifting, aren't as likely to have sudden back strains and sprains. It's mostly the neglectful ones, the weekend athlete and occasional exerciser, who invite back miseries.

As an example, a former secretary of mine went on a picnic with her husband and three children. After they played a rousing game of softball, she went home exhausted. When she got out of her car she found she couldn't straighten her back. Her husband had to help her to bed and gave her aspirin for her pain. When she got up she found that she could straighten up and assumed she had had a little muscle spasm from the unaccustomed exercise. However, the next day she had trouble getting up from her chair. It was several moments before she could bring herself erect.

What followed was constant misery. She was examined by a number of health professionals and tried everything recommended, from sleeping on a board to an orthopedic back brace, all without improvement. She needed twelve aspirin tablets just to get through the day.

When she came to work for me she was still wearing her special back brace. Eight months later she walked into my office and told me her story and confessed that her husband had to pick her up after work every day so that she could lie down flat in the back seat going home. She was thinking of quitting work because of the constant pain aggravated by sitting and asked if there was a chance that exercise could help. I explained that we had to get the blood flowing through the muscles and get them working again. I then outlined an exercise she could do at home. I also warned her that it might feel worse before it felt better. She was ready.

The first exercise I showed her was the **One Arm Dead Lift** (the exercise I describe later in this chapter for strengthening the weak side of the back to make it even with the strong side). Because she had no weights at home, I suggested that she put a couple of bricks, weighing about 10 pounds, in a tote bag about 11 by 16 inches. I had her stand with her feet a shoulder width apart holding the weighted bag in her right hand (her left side was the painful one). Next I had her slightly bend her knees (to take the strain off her back) and lean over at the waist and lower the bag in front of her right foot. I then had her pick up the bag, straighten up and lean back slightly to the left. The next step was to place the bag in front of her left foot and repeat, alternating right to left.

The second exercise was **Side Bends** with the weighted bag. I had her put the weight in her right hand, left hand behind her head, bend from the waist to the left side, then to the right as far as it was comfortable, six times (three on each side). I then had her change the weight to her left hand, right hand behind head, and repeat six times, keeping the muscles in the midsection tensed.

She did her exercises faithfully and increased her repetitions as she progressed. After one month she was off the aspirin and after two months she had no more back pain. That was many years ago and she still has her little tote bag. Later on in this chapter, when we talk about the sacro spinal mass and the obliques, I'll repeat these exercises.

The fifties and over, which we're examining in this book, is a time when men and women face the facts of life soberly and realize why health is so important to their future and why they'd better make corrections. It is a time of looking ahead, looking back at your life, and looking closely at the life of your back. It's common knowledge that young people recover more swiftly from illness than older people. As we age our recuperative powers slow down. We can't prevent all illnesses from befalling people, but if this regimen of nutrition, exercise, and common sense can prevent some of these ailments from coming your way, then this book will have been worth the effort.

It isn't only nonathletic sitters who have back problems

in middle age. I remember an Oakland businessman, in his forties, who had such a bad sacroiliac condition he had to take to his bed two or three times a year. By the time he came to me he had been in and out of traction and was using braces and belts to support his back. He was an active, athletic man with two hobbies—sports and eating. It was the second hobby that undid the first. He didn't realize that his big protruding stomach was one of the causes of his problem. The bones in your spine are held in place by muscles, ligaments, and tendons. If you don't have good stomach and back muscle development it can throw off the alignment in the spine and cause pain.

The first thing I did was to have him quit exceeding his feed limit and trim down that midsection. Then I gave him exercises for the stomach and lower back. Here was a sometimes weekend sports participant who didn't believe in regular systematic exercise. He thought he was invincible until he continued to have chronic back problems. After getting into a regular exercise program, I'm pleased to say that he went on into his sixties a healthy content-ed man.

In the beginning of this chapter I listed the muscles that help strengthen and support your lower back. If I were asked to recommend some simple all-purpose exercises for those areas, they would be the following. (Assuming, of course, that your medical examination permits such activ-ity. Check with your doctor before attempting these exer-cises.)

The **Psoas Muscle** (from the part of your low back that faces forward and connects to the thigh bone; bends or raises your leg at the hip):

**Knees to Chest Exercise:** Sit on a straight chair, raise and bend your knees. Bring your right knee into your chest and try to touch your nose. Hold for 10 seconds, and bring back to original position. Now bring your left knee to your chest, hold for 10 seconds, and then back to the original position. Alternate legs. For a more advanced stretch, lie flat and keep the opposite leg straight as you bring your knee to your chest. Start out with 5 on each leg and depending on your condition work up to 15. Breathe deeply. Exhale as your stomach muscles contract (when you bring your knee to your chest) and inhale as your leg comes down.

The **Gluteus Maximus** (the big muscles in your hips):

**Alternate Leg Lifts Face Down:** Lie face down on a firm surface with a pillow under your hips. With your knee straight, lift your right leg up and hold for a count of 5 and repeat with your left leg. Start with 5 repetitions and work up to 15. Breathe deeply.

The **Leg Extensions to the Back** exercise that I described in Chapter 11 is also a good one for this area.

The **Sacro Spinal Mass** (muscles in the lumbar region that support either side of the spine):

**Cat Stretch:** Get down on your hands and knees. Let your stomach and back fall toward the floor and lift your head. Now put your chin on your chest and arch or hunch your back toward the ceiling.

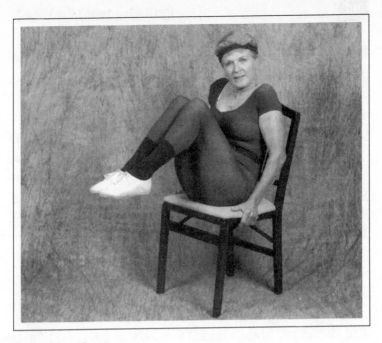

**Knees to chest**

**Knees to chest**

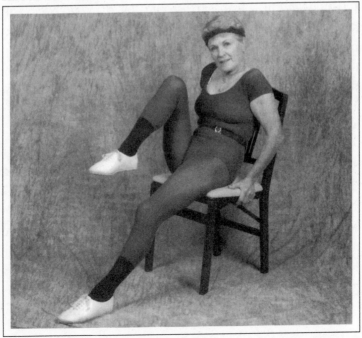

**Pelvis Tilt:** Lie on your back, knees bent, arms straight, palms down. Now lift your hips off the floor and hold for a count of 2 and repeat 2 or 3 times. Work up to 10.

**One Arm Dead Lift:** Use a small weight, perhaps a dumbbell or a used bleach bottle. Fill the bleach bottle with water to the weight you want to work with. With the weight in your right hand, arm straight, bend your knees, lean over at the waist, and lower the weight in front of your right foot. Then come erect, leaning slightly to the left. Do the same using the opposite hand. As you progress, consider a heavier weight. Start with 1 or 2 reps on each side and progress to 10.

The **Erectus Abdominus** (the abdominal or stomach muscles):

**Crunches:** On a firm surface, lie flat on your back with knees bent. Let your arms rest on your chest or, if you are more advanced, join your hands behind your head and try to sit up, or roll up until your shoulder blades are off the floor. (Do not try to sit up all the way.) Lie down and repeat. Exhale as you come up, inhale as you lie down. Start with 5 reps and increase to 15.

The **Obliques** (the muscles in the sides of the waist that make you bend from side to side):

**Side Bends:** Standing up or even sitting in a chair (without arms), bend from your waist to the right side then to the left. Start with a count of 10 (5 on each side and increase gradually). As you become stronger, add a book or a dumbbell for resistance. Caution: Never use jerky movements in

**Side bends**

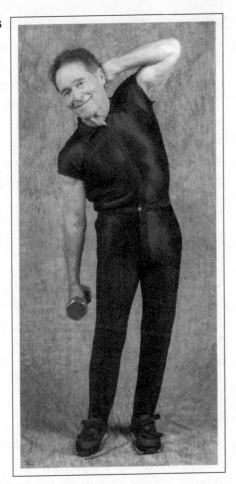

any of your exercises. A variation of the side bend when standing is to try to touch the back of your opposite knee.

Also try the **Windmill** Exercise I described in Chapter 10 on page 62.

Stretching is very important to your back. Keep in mind we are fighting gravity, so the vertebrae get compressed when we sit and stand too much. The pads between the vertebrae, the intervertebral discs, are just like little shock absorbers. As you get older and from lack of exercise these discs shrink down so they are not protecting the vertebrae. This is where the stretching, bending, and turning exercises are helpful. If you have a horizontal bar in your home, hang for 30 seconds or so and feel the stretch in your spine. If you do not have one, try standing against a wall and slowly climb the wall with your hands trying to touch the ceiling. You can also hang from the top of the door frame, and stretch.

A few do's and don'ts to help prevent back pain:

1. Do not sit in one position too long. Sitting is stressful. Move about and stretch. Keep your blood circulating.

2. Do not sit or stand in a slumped or slouched position. Avoid overstuffed furniture when you sit. Choose seats that support your lower back.

3. Use good posture at all times. Stand tall, walk tall. Always be conscious of your waist. Make it a habit to tighten your abdomen.

4. When you lift anything substantial, squat, bend with your knees, and lift with your legs, not your back. (The leg muscles are the strongest in the body.) Never lift or twist with your legs straight and avoid lifting heavy objects above shoulder level. Hold objects close to the body when lifting.

5. Try not to carry unbalanced loads.

6. When you drive, adjust the seat to keep knees and hips level. Do not strain to reach for the pedals. Keep your waist pulled in.

7. If you have a back problem, check with your physician regarding a good back support or a specially designed

pillow to help you preserve the natural curves in your spine. If a chair or car seat does not fit, use a support cushion, rolled pillow, or even a rolled up towel behind your back.

8. Sleep on a firm mattress and avoid sleeping on your stomach.

9. If for some reason you should strain your back, call your doctor and apply an ice pack (for approximately 15 minutes) several times a day. Do not place ice directly on your body. Put it in a plastic bag and cover with a towel or cloth.

10. Avoid running on hard surfaces; instead, get into a walking program. Water exercises and swimming are good for your back because they are non–weight bearing.

11. Don't try to bend over with your legs straight.

12. Listen to your body. If your back hurts, stop and rest.

I hope you'll never have to exclaim "Oh, my aching back!" again.

## Chapter 15

# The Battle of the Bulge: Your Waistline Is Your Lifeline

Time was when the girl was slim and trim; today the matronly body bulges out. Time was when the boy was lithe and limber; today the man has begun to droop over at the waist.

Most people kid themselves when they look in the mirror because they see themselves from the neck up. Use a full-length mirror for constructive criticism. Stand nude before your mirror. Don't suck in your breath. Don't tighten your stomach muscles, buttocks, or biceps. Turn around slowly and examine yourself full-face, profile left, profile right, and rear view. Be honest, what do you see? Fullness around the eyes? Biscuit-dough skin that is starting to hang and sag? Perhaps a double chin and two or three inches of loose flesh at your waist? How about the underside of your arms? Have the sands of time shifted?

Those are the things that make you look older. Your weight may be just right for your height. You may not have a weight problem, but just a little thickening all over, a telltale sign of middle age. An artist once drew a picture for me of identical twin girls. On one he sketched a double chin. Just that one addition made her look ten years older than her identical sister. That's what a bulge can mean to any of us over 50.

Americans unfortunately seem quite susceptible to bulges. "Middle-age spread," "the corporation," "cellulite." I use these terms to bring home the fact that we must fight against this problem with exercise and proper nutrition.

Fat accumulates on parts of the body where there's least activity. When there is no activity, fat likes to hibernate and find a place where it can go to sleep. That's where its friends, the other fats, gather to hang, sag, and droop. Fat is also like a river—it will flow to whatever part of the body that has the least resistance.

Fat's not funny. Fat kills. It kills people of all ages. It kills beauty, it kills desire, and even kills some people's social activities and self-esteem. Fat and the bulges it causes have come to be associated with couch potatoes. Individuals who really aren't old at all, feel older than they are and often dress in baggy-looking clothes to hide their neglect. Often that's what happens when you let yourself go.

My friend Richie Ornstein was in just such a state. He cleaned his plate at every meal, stuffed himself with junk food between meals, and was 50 pounds overweight. He went on diet after diet but could never stay on them because he was always hungry. One day when we were talking I explained to him that he could actually eat off his weight by eating three meals a day or even five meals a day if he would only put the proper fuel in his mouth and exercise regularly. I told him that anything in life is possible but he

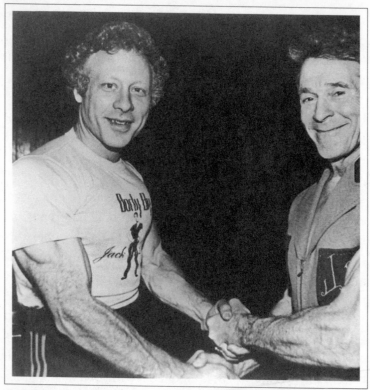

**Former New York detective, Richard Ornstein, after Jack's exercise and nutrition program trimmed 50 pounds off his body and put him back in shape. Richard is the producer of the Joe Franklin show.**

had to make it happen and to set a goal for himself and go for it. He did, and today he is in the fitness business and is out inspiring others. Recently he wrote this note to me in hopes that he might inspire some of you: "I lost over 50 pounds in about two months and over 10 inches from my waistline. I learned that there was no such word as impossible in the LaLanne dictionary if you believe in yourself and set reasonable long and short term goals. Here are some of my do's and don'ts:

- Don't eat until you are stuffed. Practice leaving some food on the plate.
- Don't give in to temptation when you go to parties. Use common sense and substitute the junk foods with salads and healthy food.
- Don't reward yourself with junk food because you have lost some weight or inches. Reward yourself with clothes or something you can't eat.
- Eat foods in their natural state and as many varieties as you can.
- Modify your lifestyle to fit your new way of taking care of yourself. You didn't put on the extra pounds over-night, so don't expect them to go away instantly. Be patient and you will reach your goals.

"So many people say they are going to start an exercise program on Monday but somehow Mondays come and go. Don't procrastinate. START NOW for a new you. As your waistline shrinks your confidence will grow. I have kept the extra pounds off for over fifteen years, if I can do it, anyone can. Thanks, Jack, for inspiring me to perspire!"

Then there are people who are proud of the fact that they haven't done much exercise over the years yet they still weigh the same as when they got out of college. "How many inches have you put on your waist since then?" was my question to them. "Oh, maybe four or five inches," is often the answer. They don't seem to realize that they have lost youthful muscle tissue and replaced it with just plain fat. The scales deceive us but the tape measure doesn't. Your waistline is your lifeline and if you want to get it down, you have to eat and exercise it off. Your waist is four sided: You have the front, two sides, and the back, and all sides need exercise. The more you exercise the faster you're going to burn up the calories. Also, when you are burning these extra calories it is important to keep your daily caloric intake to about 1,500 calories or less. Strive to get your waistline down to what it was in your prime.

Women seem to have more of a problem with the bulges on their hips and thighs. Men seem to complain more about the fatty tire around the middle.

I have already given you some exercises that help control the Battle of the Bulge and will give you more as we go along. Anything cardiovascular, fifteen to twenty minutes or more, three or four times a week, such as walking, running, swimming, bicycling, and even working out with weights (if you don't rest between sets) burns up fat. The harder you breathe, the more oxygen you take into your bloodstream and the faster you burn up fat. It's very similar to your fireplace: The more air you give your fire the faster it burns. I like to think of us as combustion engines, the more we eat and the less we exercise the slower the fat burns, but the less we eat and the more we exercise the faster we burn and lose the fat. The less fat you have to carry around the more energy you are going to have. Every pound of excess fat puts a needless strain on your heart.

The body is truly a wonderful thing. The harder it works the stronger it becomes. Each time the heart beats it pumps oxygen and nutrients through the arteries to all parts of the body. Your heart rate indicates how efficiently your heart is working. Your resting heart rate is determined when your heart is at rest (it is best to take it just upon waking in the morning). The most common spot is on the wrist, although, it can be taken at the neck, under the corner of your jaw, or below the ear. To take your pulse, place your forefinger and your middle finger on your pulse, check the second hand on your watch and count the pulse beats for fifteen seconds and multiply by four. The average person has a resting pulse rate of about 70.

If you are about to exercise aerobically, your pulse can be your guide to stay within 60 to 70 percent of your maximum heart rate.

How do you determine your maximum heart rate? Start with the number 220, subtract your age, and the result is your maximum heart rate. Say you're 50 years old; subtract 50 from 220, which puts your maximum heart rate at 170. It is not advisable to work out to your maximum, however, except perhaps when doing a stress test under a doctor's supervision. You want to stay in a safe range of exertion that is approximately 60 to 70 percent of your maximum heart rate. Thus, if your maximum is 170, 60 percent of 170 is 102, 70 percent would be 119. So between 102 and 119 heartbeats per minute is a safe range where you are strengthening the heart and not overstressing it.

It is a good idea to monitor your heart rate when you are working out. Record it, and watch the progress. Work toward the goal of lowering your pulse rate. As it lowers you are saving all those heartbeats and your heart is working more efficiently.

Let's start out with an easy exercise:

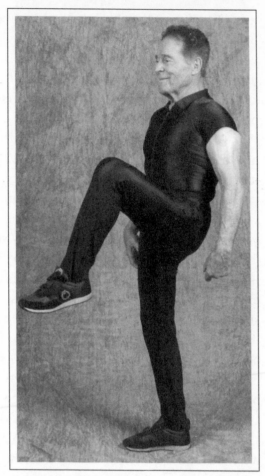

**Marching in place**

**Marching in Place:** As you march, bring each knee up as high as possible swinging your arms as you march. Count to 60, take your pulse and check it with the formula I have just given you. Is it in the target zone of 60 to 70 percent of your maximum heart rate? As you advance you can break into running in place. To make your exercise more enjoy-able, turn on some lively music.

All of the exercises I have given you so far will help you win the Battle of the Bulge. (Refer to the exercise chart on pages 183–86.) Remember the mirror doesn't lie. When you look into it, imagine how you would like to look. Every time you work out and every time you put something into your mouth, pretend you are sculpturing your body to get to your objective. And be aware, too, that what you eat today is walking and talking tomorrow.

# Chapter 16

# Aches and Pains

A stream of aches and pains seems to encompass us as we get older. Constipation, sleeplessness, tired, aching hands and feet, stiff knees and joints, indigestion, nervous tension, shortness of breath, high blood pressure, and chronic lethargy. One or many of these symptoms can cause depression, boredom, dissatisfaction, and discontent because most people feel these are just signs of old age and nothing can be done about it. So what do we do? We look for crutches such as sleeping pills, pep pills, laxatives, high blood pressure pills, antacids, pain pills, alcohol, cigarettes, and so on.

The President's Council on Physical Fitness has been telling us for years that many of our aches and pains come from lack of physical activity.

Aches and pains don't have to slow down your lifestyle after 50. Your later years can be some of the most productive and pleasant ones of your life. You are never too old to improve. Our body is the only machine in creation that is continuously repairing itself. It is constantly creating new cells from the food we give it and constantly maintaining tone when we help it along with proper exercise and nutrition, no matter how old we are.

Let's look into some of the distressing problems that might be plaguing you and show you how they might be relieved. Constipation is one of the most common. Some people seem to be troubled all their lives by irregularity. Fortunately, they are in the minority. For most people the problem creeps up gradually and becomes noticeable later in life. The reason is that regularity is attuned to general health. Nervous tension may interfere with it. Lack of liquids in the diet, leading to the formation of hard stools, may also bring it on. So does a lack of physical activity. In some people's diet, it's a lack of sufficient bulk-forming food like fresh fruits, whole grains, and raw vegetables that causes constipation. Stay away from foods that are binding, such as cheese, bakery goods, and those with a lot of fat. Eat foods in their natural state as much as possible. Make your salads with at least five to ten finely chopped, raw vegetables. Undercook your vegetables. The new electric steamers are great for just that purpose. Drink plenty of liquids, particularly those eight glasses of water a day between meals. Add to these exercises like the Magic Fives I gave you in Chapter 11 and you're doing a lot to alleviate the laxative habit. You don't have to take my word for it, check with your doctor. He or she knows your condition best.

Another intruder that plagues our good health is sleeplessness. Insomnia is much like constipation in that stress or nervous tension can bring it on or aggravate it until there's almost no coping with it. That's why you find sleeping pills in so many medicine cabinets next to the laxatives. Too much stress and too little activity.

If you are troubled with on-going insomnia, see your physician, as it might require therapy. I'm addressing here the temporary insomnia you might be enduring. There are a number of reasons you might be having sleep problems: loss of a job, a death in the family, traveling long distances by air, worry, trying to live in tomorrow when tomorrow isn't here yet, or too much alcohol. Insomnia can also be very deceiving. Some people think they have a sleep problem, but they don't need as much sleep as they think. Some of us get along on five hours of sleep while others can't seem to function unless they get eight to ten hours. I don't believe there is any set amount of sleep that one should have. It varies with each individual. It's how you feel the next day; if you feel rested you probably got enough sleep. To help you sleep better, take a warm bath before retiring, think positive thoughts, and reflect on beautiful things and experiences. Don't dwell on problems of the day, there isn't anything you can do about them at the moment. Don't relive the past, yesterday has gone. Postpone your decision making until the next morning and don't worry about getting to sleep. If you feel you can't sleep, get up, read a book, make yourself some herbal tea. Your diet may be lacking B vitamins, which can create mental confusion. I call the B vitamins your morale vitamins. To sleep you have to relax. Singing coaches get their students to relax before going onstage by breathing deeply and rhythmically for a few moments. Try the deep breathing exercises I described in Chapter 10 and flood your body with life-giving oxygen.

Tired, aching feet can be a big problem as we grow older. You hear about sore feet almost as much as aching backs.

In the past, style has been one of the causes of aching feet. Today people are wearing more comfortable shoes. Among them is my wife, Elaine, who wore high heels for years. Now her feet are happier and so is her lower back.

Your feet are the lowest extremity of your body. The heart has to pump blood down there and back up again. That's why the poorest blood supply is in our feet. If the lower legs do not get enough exercise, the muscles and the arteries become weak and cannot do their pumping job. Consequently, they lose their elasticity. This impairs the circulation and can cause swelling and aches and pains in the legs and feet. When you exercise the lower legs, you strengthen the muscles that do the pumping of the blood back to the heart and lungs. This helps your circulatory system become stronger and more efficient.

Here are several exercises you can do to strengthen and bring more circulation to the lower legs:

**Toe Raises:** Hold on to a chair for balance and rise up on your toes and then down. Rise up and down 8 to 10 times and work up to 15 or 20. As you progress, these can be done standing on a block of wood or a book. Place your toes on the edge of the block of wood or book and lower heels to the floor, hold for a count of 2 and rise up and down 8 to 10 times. Toe raises can also be done with your toes pointing out and pointing in.

**Heel and Toe Walk:** When you walk on your heels you are working the soleus muscle, the muscle in the shin area. When you walk on your toes you are working the gastrocnemius muscle, the muscle in the calf area of the leg. Walk around the room doing the Heel and Toe Walk. This helps bring blood to the lower extremities and increases circulation. It also stretches the tendons and ligaments.

**Rolling Pin Roll:** This exercise is easier do to without socks or stockings. Roll your feet over a rolling pin that's on the floor. Roll it back and forth. This is a good one to do while you're watching TV at the end of the day.

**Toe Grip:** This one is also easier to do without stockings. Place a large marble or small ball on the floor. Pick it up with your toes and raise your leg until it is parallel to the floor. Hold for a count of 5. You can also do this while watching TV.

Many of our joints can cause pain if we neglect and don't use them—the knees particularly because they are so vulnerable. In later years the constant stress of excess weight on your body can cause stiffness, pain, and swelling. For occasional pain you can try simple exercises, but if you have constant pain in the knees it's important to see your physician.

There is no one more aware of knee problems than I. In 1933, in my last football game in high school, I was hit in the knees and had one of the first knee operations. I was on crutches for three months and was told that I would probably never walk again. When the cast was removed atrophy had set in and my leg was shriveled and withered. I mentioned earlier that I had studied *Gray's Anatomy* all through school and had firemen and policemen working out in my backyard, keeping records of their progress similar to a thesis for a degree. I was convinced that my research and my knowledge of kinesiology would enable me to rehabilitate my knee. I was determined to walk again. Little by little I put more pressure on the leg. I began a series of exercises on a machine I designed. The machine is known today as the leg extension machine. I still have that very first machine in my home today. It was hand hammered and handmade of steel by a blacksmith in Oakland, who later went into the gym equipment business.

There is a street in Berkeley named Marin. It is one of the steepest hills in the Bay area, one mile straight up. My goal was to walk to the top one day and as I told you, I eventually reached that goal. As I've said many times, anything in life is possible if you make it happen.

Remember, your knees and your joints are like hinges. Take a hinge and let it rust and it will squeak and creak until it gets some oil. Knees often become stiff from lack of use, and exercise is the oil for our joints.

An exercise I recommend for minor knee problems and for occasional knee pain and stiffness is **Self-Resisting Leg Extensions**. Sit in a chair, feet on the floor. Cross your right ankle over your left ankle. Raise your legs slowly, and press down hard with your top leg against the bottom leg. Slowly lower your legs and repeat. Alternate legs. Start out doing each leg 4 times.

Another exercise I often use is **Leg Lifts with a Book**: Sit in a chair with your hands grasping the sides and place a book between your ankles. Now, lift your legs together, keeping the book firmly between your ankles. Hold out straight for a count of 5 and lower your legs. Repeat 4 or 5 times and work up to 10 or 15.

If we continue to exercise progressively throughout our lives and make it a habit, just like brushing our teeth, we can help ward off early signs of arthritis. Often we neglect certain parts of our body, like hands for instance. We take them for granted and in later years when they get a little stiff and sore we can't understand why. Your doctor can advise you whether you have arthritis and if exercising the hands will help. I'm sure he will say, "Exercise by all means." We really don't use the hands as much as we think and fail to use them in all ways for which they were so magnificently constructed. I have some great exercises for

**Leg lifts with a book**

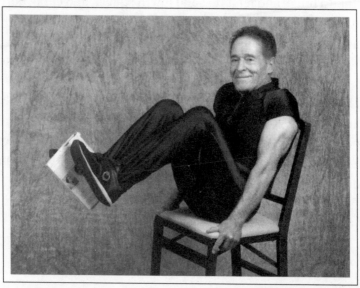

the hands, which you will probably remember from my television shows.

**Open and Close Hands:** Stand with your arms outstretched and open and close your hands as fast as possible, palms up and then palms down. Sounds easy but you'll be surprised how fast they tire. When you're finished, let them relax and shake them as hard as you can. Can you feel them tingling and the blood flowing through them? Now take your left hand and pull the fingers of your right hand back toward your arm, stretching the fingers. Repeat with the opposite hand.

**Newspaper Roll:** Take a section of newspaper (about two or three sheets) with hands on either side, roll it up and then roll in back down again. Do this several times or until your hands and arms get tired. This helps strengthen the hands and the forearms and gives you more flexibility and dexterity.

**Newspaper roll**

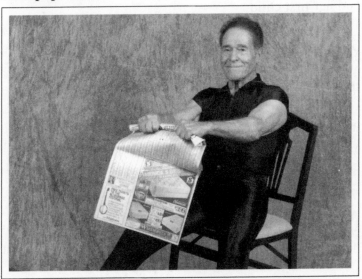

**Rubber Ball Squeeze:** Find a rubber ball that fits in your hand and squeeze it as hard as you can, first in one hand and then the other.

I gave these exercises to a friend who was discharged from the service on full disability after World War II because a hand grenade had exploded in his hand. He was faithful with his exercises and eventually became a member of the United States wrestling team and ultimately went to the Olympics.

So many of us with aches and pains that seem to settle in the joints need activity to get the blood circulating. I know men and women who have lessened the stiffening of arthritis by faithfully following daily exercise routines. I am reminded of a 45-year-old woman whose doctor recommended she come to my gym in Oakland many years ago in hopes that exercise would help her arthritis. The studio was on the second floor. She was in such pain she actually had to crawl up the stairs. Within a few months she was going out to dances with her husband and nine months later she had her first child.

When a friend of mine started feeling arthritis pains, his physician gave him some simple exercises to keep his joints supple. The exercises worked and he doesn't regret one bit the fifteen or twenty minutes a day his limbering up requires.

So far in this chapter we've discussed some of the aches and pains of aging and the crutches we must throw away. If you feel tired or low the best pepper-upper I know doesn't come in pill form, it's exercise. Here then are some simple exercises for your arms and shoulders:

**Lateral Arm Raises to Sides:** Stand straight and tall with a hardcover book in each hand. Keeping your arms straight, raise your arms laterally until they touch above your head. Slowly lower them back to the original position. Beginners do the exercise without the books. As you improve, increase the size and weight of the books. Start out with eight repetitions.

**Arm Raises to Front:** Standing, raise the books in front of you, ultimately reaching them straight above your head.

**Military Press:** Stand straight, keep that waist in. Start by holding the books out beside your ears. Now raise the books overhead, pause, and bring them back down to the same position. Using books, cans, or bottles of water as weights can provide resistance for greater effectiveness.

**Military press: 1st position**

**Military press: 2nd position**

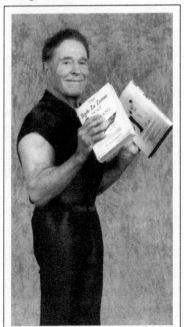

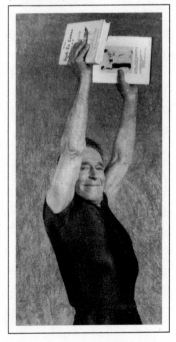

**Taut Towel:** Using a towel or a rope, grasp it firmly at both ends and pull it taut. Now pull the towel to your side and upward with your right hand while offering resistance with your left. When you bring it back down to the neutral position, pull upward with your left hand and offer resistance with your right. Repeat the process.

**Parallel Towel:** Holding a towel at both ends, pull it taut. Stand tall, waist in, arms at shoulder level. Keep your towel parallel to the floor during this entire exercise. Pull the towel slowly to the left and resist with the right hand. Then pull the towel to your right and resist with your left hand. Repeat. Start with 4 pulls in each direction and increase as you progress.

Indigestion is another problem that seems to crop up as we get older and can make our days most unpleasant. I suspect a lot of it stems from bad eating habits like bolting down food without chewing properly and could be corrected by just changing a few habits. Of course, if it persists, by all means see your doctor. For many people, however, this discomfort is just a direct result of bad food combinations. For some it's as simple as not chewing sufficiently. Starches, such as potatoes, beans, rice, bread, and other grains must be chewed thoroughly so that they can be converted to sugar by the saliva. Your stomach doesn't have teeth; the job must be done with the molars in your mouth. Proteins, like meats, can be digested by the hydrochloric acid in your stomach.

For decades, ulcers were believed to have been caused by psychological factors such as tension, anxiety, frustration, apprehension, and fear. In 1983, a 32-year-old medical resident in Perth, Australia, Dr. Barry Marshall, believed

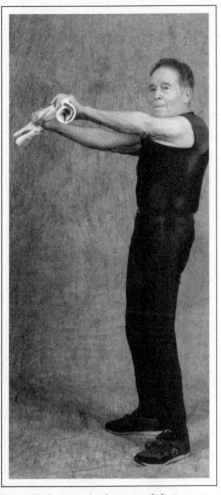

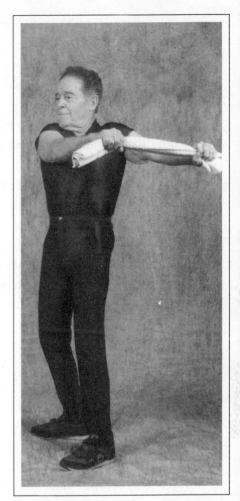

**Parallel towel: 1st position**          **Parallel towel: 2nd position**

peptic ulcers were caused by bacteria. When no one believed him, he swallowed some water filled with a bacteria
called *helicobacter*. The rest is history, though it took
almost a decade for other doctors to prove his theory. In
their attempts to prove him wrong they actually proved him
right. If the bacteria *helicobacter* is not in your stomach
you're less likely to have ulcers. Research has shown that

many people with ulcers harbor the *helicobacter pylori (H. pylori)*. When treated with antibiotics most people show no reoccurrence after twelve months. This treatment is gaining acceptance over the standard methods of treating ulcers.

Tension can also induce indigestion. Eating while worried, discussing family problems during a meal, figuring out bills that need to be paid, all may contribute to indigestion. But there are other culprits: overeating, starting the day without breakfast, not eating regularly. There are many ways of bringing on indigestion. The remedies in most cases are self-evident. You will find them all through this book.

From the time mother drops the strictly scheduled feeding care of her infant, we tend to take on detrimental eating habits. They reflect themselves in the well-being of the body. Then nature hoists all sorts of warning signals throughout our lives; decaying teeth, failing eyesight, headaches, loss of energy. We can either heed these warning signs and get medical and dental checkups or ignore them and pay the price. By our fifties, we should be intelligent enough to realize that disease or neglect does not come upon us suddenly.

One of the big storm warnings that applies to men and women in their later years is shortness of breath. Your physician can tell you if it is from a heart condition, allergies, asthma, or some presently harmless condition that could lead to heart trouble. That roll of fat around your middle might be one of the reasons for your shortness of breath. If you cut your weight down and firm up your body with exercise, you may find that you can get up a flight of stairs without breathing so hard.

Some people think it necessary to tackle problems like insomnia, aches and pains, or worry at the bottom of a bottle of liquor. This demoralizing crutch the country has come to lean upon is alcoholism. California, where I live, has become one of the biggest consumers of alcoholic beverages in the world.

There are approximately 90 calories in that alcoholic social beverage but they're all empty calories. That is, there's caloric energy but no nourishment. It even takes vitamin B from your system to digest the alcohol. If you can drink in moderation, fine, but it's the overindulgence that's the culprit and can bring on psychological lows. An apple a day is great but you wouldn't eat ten or twenty, would you? If you eat properly and exercise regularly you can probably handle moderate drinking. But if you are not keeping in shape and overindulging, it would behoove you to start a new way of life and throw away that crutch. In all things, it isn't what you do once in a while that affects the body. It's what you do most of the time.

The same would apply to that other crutch, smoking. This is one habit I would banish from all my friends if I had a magic wand. Nothing good comes from smoking. I recall an old jingle my great-uncle used to chant around the house:

> *Tobacco is a filthy weed*
> *And from the devil comes the seed.*
> *It picks your pockets, scents your clothes.*
> *And makes a chimney of your nose.*

I often mention in my lectures throughout the country that if God wanted you to smoke he would have put a chimney on top of your head.

I suspect that in this day and age we all know the serious effects of smoking. It has no beneficial effect on health. It constricts blood vessels and interferes with proper circulation. It definitely causes throat ailments and can cause lung cancer. It is also blamed for much of our coronary heart diseases. Need I say more?

I looked up the word "pain" in the dictionary and found that it is derived from the Old French word *peine,* which comes from the Latin word *poena,* which means to punish. Don't punish yourself by lack of exercise and proper nutrition. Throw away your crutches and recapture vibrant good health that you can maintain for the rest of your life. I can't do it for you, it is up to you, and you can do it.

# Chapter 17

# Be Kind to Your Heart

"Cardiovascular disease is the most common cause of death in the United States and there are about 4,000 heart attacks each day or nearly three heart attacks every minute". That figure does not come from Jack LaLanne's statistics. It comes from "The Facts," prepared by the Office of Disease Prevention and Health Promotion, U.S. Public Health Service, Department of Health and Human Services.

Those nearly three heart attacks every minute could possibly have been avoided if only those persons had heeded the advice of the American Heart Association. The association continually educates the public on how to avoid heart problems, however, few think it applies to them. Over 520,000 Americans die from heart attacks each year.

The heart is practically indestructible but many Americans continually break nature's laws and abuse it by overindulging—overeating, drinking, and smoking—and underexercising. It is like any other muscle in the body, if it isn't stressed cardiovascularly, it gets weaker. Fat infiltrates into the muscles and valves and takes away its efficiency. The heart never fails, it is the circulation going to the heart that often fails.

Probably one of the greatest phenomena in life is the human heart. In size, it is slightly larger than a fist. In shape, it is somewhat like a pear, with the larger end directed downward to the left. It is not a delicate organ, it is a powerful, hollow muscle divided by a wall down the middle into two main divisions, right and left. Each side has two chambers, the upper chamber is called the atrium, and the lower chamber the ventricle, which work together as a unit.

The blood flowing to the heart enters the right atrium (from the veins), which pumps the blood down to the right ventricle. The right ventricle pumps the oxygen-poor blood into the lungs, where it gets rid of waste gas (carbon dioxide) collected from body tissues. It then picks up fresh oxygen to carry to the other side of the heart, the left atrium, which pumps the new oxygen-rich blood to the left ventricle, sending it through the main artery (the aorta). The blood is then delivered to nourish all parts of the body, including the brain, organs, muscles, and tissues. The veins then bring the blood back to the heart and the process starts all over again.

Hopefully you can see now why I am so enthusiastic about

- deep breathing, which gives you fresh oxygen,
- posture, which helps keep our organs in proper position,
- exercise to keep the blood vessels open, and
- proper nutrition to manufacture pure blood.

Nearly all of us start life with a good heart. It was designed by the good Lord to beat faithfully and steadily, 60 to 80 beats per minute into advanced old age. What happens in between our beginning and our end? Along with other things, we take our heart for granted. We under-exercise it and overfeed it. The average American diet consists of fats, sugars, and overprocessed foods that are full of empty calories. Excess fat clogs the arteries and impairs circulation. Would you get up in the morning and give your dog or cat a cup of coffee, a cigarette, and a donut? Of course not. Would you put water in the gas tank of your car? It wouldn't run. But many of us don't realize that our human machine needs proper fuel and exercise to nourish the body's 70 trillion cells. Exercise can also help open up the blood vessels and prevent cholesterol from forming on the vessel walls.

Some of the major signs that tell us the body is not working well are: high blood pressure, excessive body fat, high cholesterol, faulty elimination, insomnia, and depression, as well as a loss of body tone, strength, and endurance. These symptoms can be helped through regular exercise, done aerobically. As I have previously advised, it is best to check with your physician before starting an exercise program.

Being kind to your heart means being kind to you and taking charge of your health. No one else can do it for you. If you want to feel good, you are the one that has to make the effort. Make the effort but, *make haste slowly*.

I suggest a consistent **walking program**, even if it is taken up later in life. The leg muscles are the largest in the body, and when you make them work for you they can help improve your health-regulating systems. A good walking

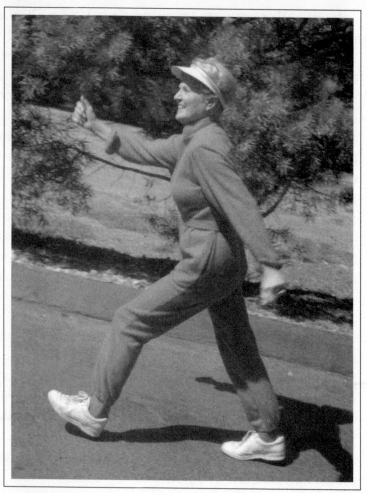

**Walk briskly**

program will also effectively make the cardiovascular system (heart, lungs, and blood vessels) perform more effectively. While walking, notice the natural movement of the arms; exaggerate this movement and you will also be helping the muscles in the upper body.

Don't wait for something to happen. Be kind to your heart now with the following tips:

1. **Exercise:** Choose aerobic activity such as I have just suggested, or swimming, bicycling, dancing, treadmill, stepper, trampoline, or even cross-country skiing. Work up to 30 minutes at least three or four times per week. Include some of the exercises that I have already given you.

2. **Lose Weight:** If you are overweight you could be a C.C. (candidate for a coronary). The more overweight you are, the higher the risk. Check with your doctor.

3. **Don't Exceed the Feed Limit:** Eat foods that are low in fat, saturated fat, and cholesterol. Fat should be no more than about 25 percent of your daily caloric intake. Eat more fruits, vegetables, and grains. Avoid processed foods. As I've always said, "Eat foods in their natural state as much as possible." Foods rich in antioxidants (beta carotene, vitamins C and E), can also help reduce the risk of heart disease.

4. **Avoid High Blood Pressure and High Cholesterol:** The higher your cholesterol level, the greater the risk of cardiovascular disease. Lower it and you lower the risk. The same goes for high blood pressure. High blood pressure has been called the "silent killer" because often there are no symptoms. It becomes more common as we age and should be checked regularly.

5. **Stop Smoking:** Heed the surgeon general's warnings about smoking. Smoking constricts the blood vessels, and the more cigarettes you smoke the higher the risk of heart disease.

6. **Avoid Stress:** Stress is not all bad for you; for instance, your muscles need to be stressed from exercise to keep them in shape. It's the stress from overwork, worry, family problems, tension, and the like that I'm talking about here. Try not to worry about the things over which you have no control.

The greatest favor you can give your heart is to exercise it and make it pump (it's the world's finest pump). Make it beat. This advice, of course, is not for those with known heart problems unless their doctor recommends it. Let him or her be the judge.

# Chapter 18

# Foods for Life

Up to this point, I've talked a good deal about the vital role exercise plays in any fitness program, with frequent suggestions that good nutrition is of equal importance to health and vitality after 50. The food you eat produces energy and helps rebuild and maintain the body. It also determines what you will look like. Exercise is the bending, turning, stretching of our bodies and the catalyst that helps metabolize and utilize the food we eat.

We are walking billboards. If we are overweight and out of shape, lack vitality and enthusiasm, we are telling the world on our billboard, "I don't care." On the other hand, if you take care of your body by giving it proper nutrition and exercise, you will exude vitality and enthusiasm. Your sign will read, "I have pride, I have discipline, I take care of this God-given body, it's my moral obligation."

The food you put in your body can be good or bad. It can be live, vital food that builds live vital bodies or it can be "junk food" that contributes to abuse, neglect, and decline of your physical condition. If you can put the proper fuel in your car, surely you can put the proper fuel in your body. One of my LaLannisms that is often quoted is "The food you eat today is walking and talking tomorrow."

I believe in the following:

- Eating foods in their natural state as much as possible.
- Eating a variety of natural foods. Too many people eat the same thing, day in and day out.
- Moderation in all things. You wouldn't eat 100 apples a day.
- Eating should be a romantic adventure.

Many of our eating habits have been handed down from generation to generation and we eat the same way our parents did. Often we create a dislike for certain foods as children, and as grownups we still harbor those dislikes. We even refuse to taste foods we think we will not like. I believe it is all controlled by your mind.

Years ago when I changed my eating habits from bad to good, I decided that I would create a dislike for any food that was deleterious to my health. I pictured this in my mind. By the same token, if it was food I didn't particularly like but would better my life, I created a liking for it.

I guess you know by now I'm a firm believer in what you put in your mouth has a lot to do with how you look and feel. Nutrition and exercise go hand in hand. You can eat perfectly, but if you don't exercise you will lose your muscle tone. On the other hand, if your diet is not perfect and you exercise vigorously, you can get by. Take athletes for instance: Many of them eat high-calorie, overprocessed foods, but they exercise so vigorously that they burn up the calories.

It's like your automobile: If you drive it 100 miles an hour the car burns up twice the amount of fuel than it does at 50. Our bodies are the same. We take in the fuel (food) that produces energy and the more we exercise, the more calories we burn.

We are hearing more and more about antioxidants. What are antioxidants? When an apple is cut and exposed to the air it starts to discolor from oxidation. The same happens with a banana; oxidation takes place, and it turns brown. Squeeze some lemon on it and the process stops. What does the lemon have in it that keeps the apple or banana from discoloring? Researchers have found that the lemon contains vitamin C, an antioxidant, which helps prevent oxidation, not only in the apple and banana but in human cells as well. As part of their function, cells make toxic molecules called free radicals (they are actually damaged cells). Free radicals attack healthy cells, and if these cells are not armed with antioxidants like vitamins C and E and beta carotene and the cofactors zinc and selenium, these free radicals can interfere with the growth of normal cells. Research is proving that eating certain foods rich in antioxidants can help block and neutralize the damaging effects of free radicals.

Researchers are also finding, from hundreds of studies, that aging is a result of increased damage from these free radicals. Evidence suggests that eating fruits and vegetables rich in beta carotene and vitamin C or taking antioxidant supplements can reduce the risk of most cancers. Also, foods rich in vitamin E may help neutralize free radicals. This may help to decrease the chance of cardiovascular disease, which is unfortunately the number one killer in America (cancer is second).

Here is a partial list of foods rich in antioxidants: carrots, broccoli, brussel sprouts, cabbage, cauliflower, spinach, beet tops, parsley, kale, squash, romaine lettuce, potato skins, and sweet potatoes. Lemons, apples, strawberries, and even olive oil fight the free radicals.

I'd like to share with you some additional foods I have found to be essential to my physical and mental well-being over the past sixty years.

*Fruits:* Bananas, apples, pears, papaya, melons, berries, oranges, pineapple, peaches, grapefruit, figs, watermelon, avocados, and prunes are just a few. As I mentioned before, moderation in all things is the watchword. If one apple at a time is good for you, 100 are not.

My friend Tom Voiss decided that he wanted to lose 50 pounds and we talked about some of the natural healthy foods he should be eating. One of the several suggestions was fresh fruit. When we were having dinner one evening he asked me why he wasn't losing more weight. I asked him what he was eating during the day. He said mostly fresh fruit. "How much?" I asked. "Oh, about ten or so per day," he answered. I explained that he was getting about 1,200 calories in just the fruit alone. I suggested he eat more salads, vegetables, and fish. At this writing he has lost 35 pounds and is truly enjoying his well-rounded diet.

*Vegetables:* Broccoli, carrots, beets and beet greens, cauliflower, cabbage, brussel sprouts, red and green peppers, mushrooms, celery, chard, collards, snow peas, snap green beans, asparagus, turnips, egg plant, sweet corn, and my three favorite squashes, zucchini, gooseneck, and summer squash. Not to forget romaine lettuce, cucumber, onions, tomatoes (if they are ripe), pumpkins, potatoes.

*Grains:* Wheat germ, bulgur, bran, oats, rye, brown rice, whole wheat, and whole grain breads, and pastas.

*Beans and Peas:* Lentils, lima, soy, kidney, pinto, garbanzo beans, and split peas.

I have homemade soup almost every day of my life. Elaine makes either lima bean, lentil, or split pea soup for me. She also makes corn chowder without using milk. Most of our soup stock is made from vegetable broth or chicken broth. Garbanzo beans and soybeans are also a great source of protein and we often use them in our salads. We also use tofu, which is made from soybean meal; it's a good source of calcium as well as protein.

*Sprouts:* Beans, peas, alfalfa, rye oats, and barley are probably the best for sprouting. Sprouts are loaded with vitamins and minerals and are low in fat. It is easy to sprout your own or you can buy most of them at the supermarket.

In a glass jar, cover with water the beans you wish to sprout. Use cheesecloth as your lid or you can buy sprouting lids at the store. Soak the beans overnight to soften. Pour off the excess water the next day, then rinse and drain the beans. Cover the jar with the cheesecloth, tilting it slightly to let the moisture out and oxygen in, and put it in a warm, dark place. Over the next two to six days rinse and drain the beans several times a day. When the sprouts have reached the desired length, place them in a warm, sunny spot. Watch for the leaves to turn a bright green, give them a final rinse, drain and, put in the refrigerator. They should stay fresh for about two weeks when tightly sealed in a plastic bag.

*Garlic:* Garlic is incredible, it has so many therapeutic properties. It has been found to help lower cholesterol and help prevent the formation of blood clots that can lead to heart attacks and strokes. Garlic also aids in combating high blood pressure and certain kinds of cancer. We use no butter in our home but instead we use olive oil and chopped garlic mixed together as a substitute.

*Fish:* Cod, halibut, sole, swordfish, salmon, and whitefish are just a few of my favorites. I don't eat any red meat, so since we live near the ocean, my diet consists mostly of fish. I keep shellfish to a minimum and eat the freshest fish available. From time to time for lunch I will have a can of water-packed tuna or water-packed sardines.

*Chicken:* It has become one of the most popular dishes in the American diet. However, the days of free range chickens are becoming fewer and fewer. With an increased demand for chicken, poultry producers feed their birds to a marketable weight much faster. Living in such close quarters waiting to go to market, the chickens do not get enough exercise and consequently become excessively plump. Therefore, I feel it is important for you to get to know your butcher to find out if your chicken is allowed to range freely.

A little cooking tip: If you cut out the fat under the skin before you cook the bird, you'll be saving yourself a lot of calories and a lot of fat. There are racks you can buy that hold the chicken upright so that the fat drips to the bottom. Skinless chicken breasts are very popular for those of us who are concerned about their fat intake. I like to add some strips to a stir-fry of veggies. Serve it all on brown rice.

*Turkey:* Many people today are buying ground turkey to replace hamburger. Unless you buy the lean variety, you could be getting as much fat as in hamburger. Make sure you read the labels for fat content. Removing the skin will also help reduce the amount of fat in the meat. Turkey is also a less expensive source of protein. Most of us think of fixing turkey only during the holidays, but it can be prepared in a variety of ways all year round. It can be barbecued, smoked, baked, ground, sliced for sandwiches, and even made into soup. Many people think you have to buy the whole turkey, but individual pieces can be bought for everyday preparation. The possibilities are endless so long as you watch the fat content.

*Red Meat:* Beef, pork, lamb, veal. Although I personally don't eat it, the red meat industry is continually developing a leaner and leaner product. Remember, everything in moderation. Most Americans eat too much protein and too much fat. Red meat is fine as long as you watch the fat content, just as you do with poultry.

*Eggs:* Eggs are probably one of the most perfect foods available. Eggs have often been criticized for being too high in cholesterol. Studies are now showing that they are not as high as previously thought and actually the egg yolk is a source of iron, choline, and inositol (research indicates that the latter two may inhibit cholesterol buildup). A whole egg has 70 calories but the egg white has only 15 calories, 7 grams of protein, and no fat. Therefore, if you eat four egg whites you get 28 grams of protein and only 60 calories. Compare this to a pound of steak, which has approximately 1,000 calories and 25 grams of protein. By eating only the egg whites you are saving yourself approximately 900 calories and still getting 28 grams of protein with no fat.

*Dairy Products:* I rarely eat dairy products but when I do I have nonfat milk or nonfat yogurt. We've been led to believe that we never outgrow our need for milk, when we actually outgrow it during the first few years of our lives. A large portion of the world's population is lactose intolerant and cannot consume milk or other dairy products. Name me one creature that drinks milk after it has been weaned. It's not that all milk is bad for you. It's the overconsumption that can take its toll by adding excessive fat and cholesterol to the diet. A common myth is that you have to drink milk to get enough calcium in your diet, but dark green leafy vegetables like Swiss chard, bok choy, and broccoli are also excellent sources of calcium. Tofu is another great source of calcium that is eaten all over the world today. Cheese, butter, ice cream, cottage cheese, and other whole milk products are the dairy foods most often consumed. If you must have milk, make sure it is nonfat milk. There are also fat-free cheeses, yogurts, and ice creams available in today's market.

*Juices:* Apple, carrot, celery, pineapple, cranberry, orange, and grapefruit are just a few. Rather than drinking coffee, tea, or sodas, why not try fresh fruit and vegetable juices? They contain no artificial colorings or flavorings and are wonderful body cleansers. Those of you who have juicers also know how delicious they can taste. Elaine's book *Total Juicing* has some great recipes for not only the juices but also for the leftover pulp.

Any discussion of foods for life must include some thought on how we eat.

Breakfast is the key. We must have a good, healthful breakfast to get going or we simply don't have the energy to face the day. When you wake up in the morning, be aware that your body hasn't had any nourishment for ten to twelve hours. Therefore breakfast should be the most important meal of the day. Also:

- Avoid between-meal snacking on empty calories
- Chew your food thoroughly so that your body can digest it easier
- Eat your meals slowly because the slower you eat the less you eat
- Eat foods in their natural state as much as possible

My friend Dr. Gale Rudolph, Ph.D., a consultant, author, and lecturer on nutrition and food science, puts it very simply: "Low fat, high fiber, think positively, and be cheerful!"

# Chapter 19

# Your Teeth

If your teeth are gone there isn't much I can offer you except a few vital suggestions for maintaining nutrition. If you have your teeth, or most of them, take every precaution to keep them.

As you certainly know by now, I am a fervent believer in the simple, natural foods Mother Nature has given us. Science would seem to bear me out that natural foods are a basis for good dental hygiene and that we should reexamine our eating habits before we lose our teeth.

The *Journal of Dental Research* reports on a study by two anthropologists into the teeth of primitive peoples. "The teeth of primitives needed no artificial methods of cleansing. The mouths of these people were naturally clean. Natural, coarse, fibrous detergent food, vigorously chewed, swept clean the fissures and sluice ways of occlusal anatomy. It was the forceful and thorough mastication of detergent foods that gave primitive groups their caries [cavity] freedom."

One dental researcher, commenting further on modern society, said, "We have gone too far in the process of refining and synthesizing foods; the elimination of the fibrous part of the food and the omission of hard, bulky foods from our diets have caused complete disuse and lack of function of the masticators apparatus." He went on to say, "This leads to an unhygienic condition of the mouth, predisposing the teeth to caries and pyorrhea. To remedy this condition, we must eliminate the cause; and this can be accomplished only by radical revision of the culinary art and manner of preparation of food." This is the message I have been preaching for over fifty years.

Take special care of your teeth now. Good oral hygiene requires effort. Make sure you have the right toothbrush. Pick one with soft, end-rounded or polished bristles and small enough to clean your back teeth as well as the front teeth. Brush twice daily to keep bacteria from multiplying. Floss daily with waxed or unwaxed floss. Flossing removes plaque between your teeth and helps massage your gums. See your dentist at least once or twice a year for a check-up and cleaning. Too many people neglect their teeth and then they can't understand why suddenly they're confronted with gum disease. Gum disease is caused by plaque that turns to tartar. If left to build up it can irritate your gums and create pockets that can destroy the tissue and bone supporting your teeth.

Not only plaque, but the overconsumption of sugar also affects the teeth. A good example of this is our son Dan, who at 13 years of age took to chewing gum. I tried to explain to him that the sugar in the gum could affect his teeth and cause cavities. I don't think he believed me until one day he complained of a severe toothache. We took him to our dentist and found out that in the six months since Dan's last check-up his mouth was full of cavities. The dentist explained to him that if he hadn't come in when he did he could have lost all of his teeth. Dan then admitted that he was consuming at least five packs of gum a day. Needless to say, his gum-chewing days were over, and since then his visits to the dentist for check-ups and cleaning have been every three months. That was thirty-two years ago and Dan hasn't had a cavity since.

I'm not saying that sugar in moderation is going to hurt anyone, but it is the overconsumption of it that presents the problem. Too much sugar actually rotted out my baby teeth. My mother finally confessed this to me in later years after she became interested in nutrition. As a baby when I would cry or make a fuss, she would put sugar and cornstarch in a cloth, dip it in water and I would suck on it. That became my pacifier. As years passed, any time she wanted to reward me it would be with a piece of candy, cake, cookie, or ice cream. I actually became addicted to sugar until the age of 15, when I heard Paul Bragg speak at the Oakland City Women's Club. I made up my mind in one night to change my eating habits, as Dan did when he quit chewing gum.

If you find that you have a sweet tooth, look for substitutes such as fresh fruits and make sure you are supplementing your diet with B complex, vitamins C and E, calcium, and the antioxidants we talked about in Chapter 18.

Your teeth can be a warning sign that something is not quite right with your body. Heed those warning signs. It's never to late to do something about it.

"Be true to your teeth or they will be false to you."

# Chapter 20

# Blood Sugar

Do you remember the old saying "My get up and go has got up and went"? That's what happens when your blood sugar is low. You actually feel as if the river of life has been siphoned out of you. It's the old disease I talked about so many times on my television shows—Pooped-out-itis.

The key to energy is your blood sugar. When your blood sugar is up you can conquer the world and when it's down you just can't seem to push your way out of the blues. Why is this and what can we do about it?

Your blood sugar is determined by the use of energy in the food you eat. When foods are digested they must be converted to a simple sugar (glucose), the body's source of energy. This glucose then goes into the blood stream, where some of it is taken up immediately and used for energy. The rest is stored in the liver and muscles as a substance called glycogen, or as fat. When you exercise aerobically, glycogen is released and turned back into glucose to furnish energy. The regulator for converting sugar is insulin, which is produced in the pancreas. Insulin controls the rate at which glucose is removed from the blood and stored. It is vital that this release stays moderately even because if too much glucose is in the blood the body's chemical balance can be disrupted, and if there is too little, the body is robbed of energy.

When you have a sugary snack, a junk food meal, or an alcoholic drink, the body floods the system with excessive insulin and you feel a big burst of energy for a while and then a letdown. The reason for this letdown is that the flood of insulin is so great that it overpowers and stores the sugar too fast, often as fat. It's the classic afternoon slump. Often you feel the need for another rush so you turn to caffeine (coffee, tea, or cola) or another snack. Up and down, up and down. This overworking of the pancreas may eventually lead to adult onset diabetes or reduced insulin production.

On the other hand, when you ingest complex carbohydrates (beans, corn, potatoes, wheat, and whole grains), they are broken down slowly in digestion and released slowly into the blood. Then insulin reacts evenly and energy is maintained over a period of time. You'll experience fewer slumps and there will be no need to keep eating high calorie or fatty foods to maintain energy.

Exercise also aids in the digestion and assimilation of nutrients, therefore keeping energy levels even and up longer. You will also get the most use out of the calories you eat. Exercise promotes your body's ability to make good use of insulin and assists in fat loss.

It all comes back to proper nutrition and exercise. Plan proper meals at the right time. Pay attention to calories and losing body fat. Eat more fiber to assist in lowering cholesterol levels. Eat less sugar, it has lots of calories, no vitamins and minerals or food value. It plays havoc with your glucose level and with your insulin production. Eat less animal fat, it leads to heart problems and high blood pressure and is implicated in many cancers. Eat less salt, which also leads to high blood pressure and causes water retention as well as bone loss. All these hints will help you to a happier, healthy life.

# Chapter 21

# Supplements After 50

If I were persuasive enough to change every one of the eating habits you formed in your lifetime but failed to mention the importance of food supplements in your daily diet, I would consider my job only half done. In this day and age I feel that men and women who fail to supplement their daily diet with vitamins and minerals are only going partway toward peak health and vitality after 50.

No two of us eat quite the same foods or have the same digestive and assimilative powers, or the same tastes or dietary needs. I can't say to you, "Take this vitamin or this mineral," but I can tell you some of the supplements that have been best for me and recommend that you see your family health professional for advice on what supplements to take.

## The Vitamin Story

Vitamins are tiny organic substances existing in the food from plants and animals. Plants can manufacture their own vitamins but only some animals can synthesize some vitamins. Did you ever wonder why pet food manufacturers don't make "high in vitamin C" dog food? Your dog makes his own vitamin C. Although also of the animal kingdom, we humans do not. We have to get ours from the plants and animals we eat, or from dietary supplements. Supplements are also derived from living plants and animals unless they are made synthetically. I believe these micronutrients are necessary for proper growth and vitality and to regulate bodily functions.

Vitamins were discovered shortly after the turn of the century when researchers sought the reasons why some people (notably sailors deprived of fresh fruits and vegetables) developed diseases like beriberi, rickets, and scurvy. One of the first men to realize that there might be some relationship between disease and diet was Kanehiro Takaki, surgeon general of the Japanese navy. In 1882 he added meat and vegetables to his crews' diet and reduced the number of beriberi cases. A British naval officer found that his sailors didn't get scurvy if their diets were supplemented with citrus fruits. Around 1900 a Dutch medical officer discovered that people who ate polished white rice developed beriberi and those who ate the whole brown rice did not. Researchers found that there were "accessory food factors" that were essential for growth and development. A Polish chemist, Casimir Funk, coined the word "vitamine," *vita* (life) and *amine* (group of organic compounds), trying to isolate the anti-beriberi factor from rice hulls. Worldwide vitamin research has continued ever since.

On September 15, 1993, the *Journal of the Cancer Institute* announced that a five-year study was conducted by U.S. and Chinese scientists of 30,000 residents of north China. The scientists ascertained that vitamins, particularly beta carotene, vitamins C and E, and selenium can help reduce cancer deaths. The exact amounts of vitamins needed by the body are not yet known. Medical science has set up only the known minimum daily requirements (MDR), and recommended dietary allowance (RDA). Since nutrition is a rapidly growing science, new discoveries are being made all the time.

The late Linus Pauling, two-time Nobel Prize–winner, began investigating vitamin C and its relationship to the common cold over 30 years ago. Its role in heart disease and strokes is now also being studied. During this period the medical community was skeptical of these findings. Now it is taking a harder look. Researchers are finding links between vitamin C and cancer, vitamin E and heart disease, as well as between other vitamins and disease. Dr. Pauling (along with other researchers) believed that vitamins had a positive effect on the immune system. It is vital to keep your immune system working efficiently because it is your defense against foreign invaders.

I believe that the young as well as the old need to supplement their diets. The young, although active, are prone to fast food establishments, the older adults because they are less active, don't digest and absorb their food sufficiently. Many have a tendency to ease up on their exercises and become lax in regular balanced meals.

I view vitamins and minerals as an insurance policy for my diet and have been taking them for the past sixty years. Although I try to eat foods in their natural state as much as possible, I do not always know where they have been grown, if the soil was fertile, or how long the foods have been stored in the market or restaurant. We all have a number of insurance policies (home, automobile, earthquake, fire, life), so I consider vitamins and minerals added health insurance.

Vitamins are divided into two groups: fat soluble (the ones dissolved in fats, such as A, D, E, and K), and water soluble (those dissolved in water, among these the B vitamins and C). As vitamins were discovered, researchers often named them for the letters of the alphabet. There were overlaps in transcontinental research; therefore some letters were eliminated (like F) and others added ($B_2$, $B_6$, $B_{12}$, etc.).

*Vitamin A:* (Fat soluble) The first vitamin discovered and named in an alphabetical system. Can be obtained from both animal and plant sources. Studies suggest that obtaining vitamin A from beta carotene, rather than animal sources, gives you the most protection. Beta carotene is found in some fruits and in dark green and orange vegetables like carrots, sweet potatoes, collards, winter squash, spinach, kale, broccoli, cantaloupe, and apricots. It stores easily in the body and does not need to be taken every day. It is also known as an antioxidant that helps prevent cancer and lower the risk of heart disease. Vitamin A also aids in eye and skin disorders.

*B Vitamins:* (Water soluble and cannot be stored in the body) When first discovered, the B vitamins were believed to be just one vitamin. Now, more than 15 B vitamins have been isolated; the essential ones are listed here:

- *Vitamin $B_1$:* (Thiamin) Whole grains, most vegetables, potatoes, beans, liver, brewer's yeast and lean meats are sources of $B_1$. Helps release energy from food and metabolizes carbohydrates. Helps heart and nervous system to function properly. Deficiency disease is beriberi.

- *Vitamin B₂:* (Riboflavin) Eggs, milk, fish, lean meats, poultry, leafy green vegetables, liver and yeast are sources of $B_2$. Promotes tissue repair, healthy skin, hair, and nails.
- *Vitamin B₃:* (Niacinimide or Niacin) Lean meat, fish, poultry, eggs, beans, seeds, whole grains, liver, and brewer's yeast are sources of $B_3$. Helps maintain healthy skin, increases circulation, helps in the absorption of proteins and carbohydrates. Also helps keep your nervous system healthy.
- *Vitamin B₅:* (Pantothenic Acid) Found in wheat germ, whole wheat, bran, chicken, nuts, green vegetables (i.e., broccoli), kidney, liver, and brewer's yeast. Helps develop central nervous system. Cell and energy builder. Metabolizes carbohydrates and fatty acids.
- *Vitamin B₆:* (Pyridoxine) Whole grains, meat, most vegetables, sunflower seeds, beans, wheat germ, liver, and brewer's yeast. Needed for healthy teeth and gums, blood vessels, nervous system, and red blood cells.
- *Vitamin B₁₂:* (Cobalamin) Mostly obtained from animal sources: liver, kidney, heart, eggs, milk and milk products. Essential for proper development of red blood cells. Helps proper function of nervous system. Helps increase energy.

Other members of the B complex family are:

- *Biotin:* Included in most B complex supplements. Fruits, nuts, egg yolks, milk, kidney, beef liver, and brewer's yeast are sources of biotin. Energy builder and metabolizer. A deficiency is extremely rare.
- *Inositol:* Obtained from lentils, lima beans, green leafy vegetables, wheat germ, peanuts, cabbage, heart, liver,

and brewer's yeast. Helps metabolize fats and cholesterol.

• *Folic Acid:* Found in green leafy vegetables, beans,
torula yeast, and liver. Helps to absorb other B vitamins. Needed for production of red blood cells. Very
important for pregnant women

• *PABA:* Sources are whole grains, rice, bran, wheat
germ, kidney, liver, and brewer's yeast. Helps form
folic acid and utilizes protein.

• *Choline:* Obtained from green leafy vegetables, egg
yolks, wheat germ, heart, liver, and yeast. Works with
inositol to utilize fats and cholesterol. Helps control
cholesterol buildup.

I try to make sure I get all the B vitamins daily because,
1) they are not stored in the body, and 2) they are like a
chain, if one link is missing you've broken the chain. If you
take only vitamins $B_1$ and $B_6$ you are not getting all the B
complex vitamins. If you take too much of one it could give
you a deficiency in the other. I believe that when taken in
their entirety, one complements the other. Both liver from
animals and yeast from plants contain B complex and were
listed repeatedly as good sources.

Many of you may have heard about some of my swimming feats: *At age 60:* swam from Alcatraz in San Francisco Bay to Fisherman's Wharf towing a thousand-pound
boat, without a wet suit and with my hands and feet shackled. *At age 70:* towed 70 people in 70 boats a mile and a
half in Long Beach (California) Harbor, also with my
hands and feet shackled. Now what has this got to do with
vitamins?

Years ago I read a report where two groups of guinea
pigs were tested for their swimming ability. One group was

given liver and yeast, the other none. The group that did not take the liver and yeast swam about fifteen to twenty minutes, the liver and yeast group swam up to one-and-a-half hours. Well, I figured, I am of the animal kingdom, if it works for them it should work for me—and it did. I started supplementing with the de-fatted liver and yeast tablets and sincerely feel that they helped me endure the stress of the cold water and gave me the stamina to accomplish my feats.

Read the labels on B complex vitamins and you should find that they contain the B vitamins listed above: $B_1$, $B_2$, $B_6$, $B_{12}$, niacinimide, folic acid, panathenic acid, (calcium pantothenate), biotin, choline, inositol, and PABA (para aminobenzoic acid).

B vitamins are also known as the "morale" vitamins because of their effect on the nervous system and mental behavior.

*Vitamin C:* (Ascorbic Acid) Antioxidant, known to help reduce the risk of cancer. Cannot be stored in the body, so you need to obtain it every day. Probably America's most popular vitamin. Sources are citrus fruits, berries, green leafy vegetables, sweet peppers, tomatoes, cabbage, potatoes. Essential for sound bones and teeth. Needed for tissue metabolism and wound healing. Builds up the immune system and fights infections. Researchers are finding that vitamin C also helps in the treating of diabetes, high blood pressure, arthritis, cataracts, male infertility, and possibly AIDS. It is also well known as a fatigue fighter, protector against stress, and a cholesterol-lowering agent.

Ester C ascorbate was introduced into the market in 1988

and a patent was issued in 1989, which is the first patent ever granted for a vitamin C product. The manufacturer claims it can be absorbed into your system twice as fast and excreted twice as slowly as ordinary vitamin C.

*Vitamin D:* Known as the sunshine vitamin. Ultraviolet rays act under the skin and in the kidneys to produce vitamin D. However, you know very well that too much sun is harmful to your skin. Obtained from sardines, salmon, tuna, fish liver oils, and dairy products. Essential for calcium and phosphorus metabolism for strong bones and teeth. Taken with vitamins A and C, may aid in preventing colds.

*Vitamin E:* An active antioxidant, defends against free radicals. Stored in the body for only a short time, similar to vitamins B and C. Best sources are wheat germ and wheat germ oil, vegetable oils, nuts, leafy greens, and whole grain cereals. Helps maintain heart and skeletal muscles and cuts down the risk of heart disease. Helps in healing wounds and aids in resisting infection. Believed to improve oxygenation and helps slow down the aging process.

*Vitamin K:* Needed for normal blood clotting. Green leafy vegetables are the main source.

If you want to learn more about vitamins you may want to read the newly revised *Vitamin Bible* by Earl Mindell, *Jane Brody's Nutrition Book, The Doctor's Complete Guide to Vitamins and Minerals* by Mary Ann Eades, M.D., *The Right Dose* by Patricia Hauseman, M.S., and *The Complete*

*Book of Vitamins*, put out by the editors of *Prevention* magazine, to name a few.

## The Mineral Story

So much emphasis is put on vitamins today, but minerals are equally important to our general health and needed for the growth and maintenance of the body. Our bodies cannot manufacture minerals, they have to come from our environment. Our environment may not be able to give us all the minerals to satisfy our metabolic needs. People living inland didn't get iodine from seafood and developed goiters. Refining grains reduces trace elements like zinc and chromium. In many farming areas the soil is depleted of minerals, and on and on. Many women become tired and anemic from a lack of dietary iron. For these reasons many health professionals recommend supplements as added insurance.

Since the day I attended that health lecture when I was 15, I have always believed that you can't improve on Mother Nature. When I began to study vitamins and minerals over sixty years ago it was like living in the Dark Ages. People laughed and made fun of me because I was eating natural foods in their natural state. Now we are living in the age of enlightenment, and it seems that every day researchers are discovering that fresh fruits and vegetables and natural whole grains are healthier for us than the overconsumption of sugars, fats, and overprocessed and overcooked foods. Exactly what we health nuts were preaching years ago.

Minerals can be broken down into major minerals and

trace elements categories. The major minerals, ones in which the body needs a sizable amount, include:

*Calcium:* Found in sardines, salmon, walnuts, green leafy vegetables (broccoli, kale, spinach, turnip greens), beans, lentils, figs, egg yolks, and dairy products. Known to help prevent osteoporosis, lower chances of colon cancer, help keep blood pressure low and the heart beat regular.

*Magnesium:* Almost all foods contain magnesium, a component of every cell in the body. Magnesium is a part of the enzyme that absorbs vitamin C as well as sodium, phosphorus, and potassium. Aids in building strong teeth and bones. Helps to fight depression and to maintain the nervous system. Researchers are studying the possibility of a link between heart disease and low levels of magnesium.

*Phosphorus:* Found in nearly all foods. Along with calcium, builds strong bones and teeth. Needs vitamin D and calcium for proper functioning. Your body needs twice as much calcium as it does phosphorus.

*Potassium:* Found in a great number of foods. Good sources are tomatoes, green leafy vegetables, and fresh fruits like bananas, cantaloupe, apricots, and avocados. Works inside cells to flush out body wastes and helps to maintain blood pressure.

*Sodium:* Table salt (sodium chloride), beets, carrots, artichokes, dried beef, shellfish, bacon, soy sauce and all salty foods are sources of sodium. Sodium and potassium regulate the body's water balance but too much sodium depletes potassium and can throw it off balance. This may be one of the causes of high blood pressure and water retention.

The trace elements, ones in which the body needs only small amounts, are chromium, iron, iodine, sulfur, zinc, selenium, manganese, copper, cobalt, fluorine, and molybdenum.

*Chromium:* Works with insulin to metabolize sugar and helps regulate blood sugar. Sources: brewer's yeast, shellfish, chicken, clams, and meat.

*Iron:* Helps build red blood cells to prevent anemia. Sources: organ meats, fish, nuts, eggs, spinach, asparagus, prunes, and raisins.

*Iodine:* Iodine is essential for the normal function of the thyroid gland. Kelp, seafood, and vegetables grown in iodine-rich soil are natural sources.

*Sulfur:* Found in garlic, onions, high-protein foods, beans, asparagus, and egg yolks. Known to maintain healthy skin, hair, and, nails. Also helps build enzymes and maintain normal body metabolism.

*Zinc:* Helps growth of skin, hair, and nails, metabolizes carbohydrates, maintains enzyme systems, aids in healing wounds, and assists liver to utilize vitamin A Found in whole grains, nuts, wheat germ, seafood, and brewer's yeast.

*Selenium:* An antioxidant that works with antioxidant vitamins E and C. Together they help protect our bodies from free radicals that oxidize our cells causing aging and sometimes cancer (see Chapter 18 on antioxidants). Food sources: whole grains, wheat germ, bran, kidney, liver, seafood, onions, broccoli, and nuts.

*Manganese:* Needed for development of bones and connective tissue and the utilization of food. Whole grains, nuts, dried legumes, green leafy vegetables, peas, and beets are best sources.

*Copper:* Helps to release iron to form hemoglobin and aids in the absorption of iron for energy. Assists in the utilization of vitamin C. Found in most foods, especially in dried beans, whole grains, dried fruit, prunes, organ meats, and seafood.

*Cobalt:* Researchers discovered that cobalt was an essential part of vitamin $B_{12}$. Helps to prevent anemia. Only small amounts are needed and are found in most foods, especially in grains, seeds, leafy vegetables, kidney, liver, and some seafoods.

*Fluorine:* Years ago studies of children in Colorado and surrounding states revealed that those who had a dark discoloration of their teeth had fewer cavities. Researchers found that it was due to the high amount of fluorine in the water of the area. Since then many communities in the United States have added small amounts of fluorine to their water supply. Studies show that it has reduced cavities in children at least 50 percent. Found in drinking water and some seafood, such as sardines and salmon. It is also known to help strengthen bones.

*Molybdenum:* Believed to be important for enzyme utilization, especially iron. Found in whole grains, wheat germ, legumes, eggs, nuts, seeds, and yeast.

Over 60 minerals have been identified, but the preceding lists are currently considered to be the most essential.

*Silicon, Vanadium, Nickel, and Tin:* Found to be essential for normal growth in animals and studies are under way to determine their function in humans. They are found in most foods.

Most minerals are supplied to us in the natural foods we eat, but they can be destroyed in the cooking or processing of those foods. Therefore, you should try to get your minerals in natural foods as much as possible because Mother Nature put them there in the proportions she intended us to have. It is wise, before supplementing with minerals, to know how your body absorbs them, because taking large amounts of some minerals can create deficiencies in others. Why spend money if you are not going to give your body the best chance to use what you swallow? Your nutritionist or health professional will be able to help you.

## The Enzyme Story

Enzymes are protein molecules that accelerate or catalyze the chemical reactions of living cells. These tiny chemical substances break down our food in the digestive tract so it can be absorbed into the blood. Without them digestion is retarded, food isn't metabolized and malnutrition occurs.

There are more than a thousand known enzymes, each with its own function. Some can break up sugar but are powerless against fat; fat enzymes are impotent against protein; some enzymes change sugar into glycogen and some (in the saliva) convert starch into sugar. One enzyme aids in blood clotting, another starts bodily decay. Almost all the foods we eat would be completely indigestible without enzymes.

In addition to their protein part, many enzymes contain a much smaller nonprotein group called a coenzyme. Coenzymes are made up in part of individual vitamins or minerals and are essential for enzymatic activity. Niacin, for example, is part of a coenzyme for several enzymes that have to do with the taking in of oxygen by the cells.

The important thing to remember is that *we get the enzymes we need from the food we eat or we manufacture the enzymes from the protein we eat.* We must eat properly balanced foods, natural foods in sufficient quantity. I know this is can be a problem for busy people either unaware or unconcerned with diet. But before supplementing with enzymes, let me stress again that you check with your health professional to be sure you know what your body needs.

## Chapter 22

# Macronutrients: Carbohydrates, Proteins, and Fats

The macronutrients are the major dietary fuels that make up the foods we eat. Carbohydrates, proteins, and fats are used by the body to provide energy. However, they do not supply the same amounts of energy, which is measured in units called calories. For instance, carbohydrates and proteins contain equal amounts of calories, whereas fat has twice the number of calories.

*Carbohydrates:* There are basically two kinds of carbohydrates, simple and complex. Simple is composed of molecules like a mildly sweet sugar called glucose, which is rapidly absorbed into the bloodstream and the cells carry it to all parts of the body. Glucose is the fuel used by hospitals when patients are unable to ingest enough calories on their own. Complex carbohydrates consist of simple carbohydrates joined together in long chains and include starch, cellulose, and glycogen. The carbohydrates we eat consist mostly of starch, sugar, and fiber. The starches and sugar have to be broken down by the digestive process into simple sugars in the body before they can be used as energy. On the other hand, fiber, a complex carbohydrate, passes through the body practically unchanged because we humans do not have the enzymes needed to break it down to get calories from it.

Today more and more nutritionists are encouraging us to eat more complex carbohydrates. They are probably the cheapest and most efficient source of energy and are obtained mostly from grains, potatoes, and legumes, which have to be broken down in the body to simple sugars before they can be used as energy. (See Chapter 20 on Blood Sugar.) If, however, too many carbohydrates are ingested and cannot be stored in the liver as glucose and glycogen the rest is stored as fat. Almost every article on nutrition today recommends foods high in fiber (whole grain breads and cereals) to help promote bowel regularity. Raw fruits, vegetables, and pastas are also recommended sources of carbohydrates and fiber.

*"Protein,"* wrote Dr. Lester M. Morrison a number of years ago, "is the keystone of human nutrition. It is essential for every form of life for growth, pregnancy, formation of blood, bone and every vital tissue. It is essential for the healing of wounds, the warding off of infection, the maintenance of body weight, and the conduct of vital organs and glands in the body."

To which I add that lack of protein in our diet is the culprit most often responsible for what I call chronic "pooped-out-itis," a term I use for lack of energy. Pooped-out-itis can also be traced to bad eating habits, lack of sleep, or a need for more exercise.

Proteins are the building blocks of the body. Your skin,

hair, fingernails, bones, and teeth take their basic formation in protein. Your brain, nerve tissues, muscles, organs, glands, the miles of blood vessels, and even your hormones and the hemoglobin in your red cells are of protein structure.

Medical authorities agree that normal adults and growing children require 1 gram of protein for every 2.2 pounds (equal to 1 kilogram) of body weight. This means that the average man or woman weighing 125 to 175 pounds needs 60 to 80 grams of protein daily for normal nutrition. Protein is one commodity our body does not store for future needs; we have to keep replenishing it.

Protein is comprised of a chain of amino acids, made up of molecules of carbon, hydrogen, oxygen, and nitrogen. Amino acids are divided into two groups—essential, those provided in your food, and nonessential, those not supplied by diet but manufactured in the body. There are two types of proteins, complete and incomplete. The complete proteins (meats, seafood, poultry, eggs, milk, and cheese) contain all the essential amino acids to support new tissue growth, while the incomplete proteins (nuts, seeds, peas, grains, and beans) are in insufficient amounts and need essential amino acids to make them complete. Take lentils and rice, for instance. They are not a complete protein but when you eat them together they become complete because what one is lacking the other has. If you would add an egg white to either the rice or the lentils it would also become complete because the egg complements the other. You don't necessarily have to have animal protein. Complement your protein sources; mix beans with corn or rice. I have briefly touched on the subject; your bookstore or library will have more information on macronutrients and food values.

*Fats:* They furnish twice as much fuel and energy for the body as the same amount of proteins or carbohydrates because they contain more carbon and hydrogen. The combination of fatty acids and glycerol makes up fat. The most common form of fat stored in our bodies is called a triglyceride (three fatty acids connected to one molecule of glycerol). The dominant fatty acid in the fat is what constitutes its taste and whether it will be liquid or solid.

There are three types of fats:

1. *Saturates:* Include whole milk, dairy products, butter, lard, and other animal products. In the realm of vegetable oils this group includes coconut, palm, and hydrogenated oils. This group is the most troublesome.

2. *Polyunsaturates:* They are usually liquid at room temperature. They include safflower, soybean, corn, cottonseed, sesame, sunflower oils, and most margarines.

3. *Monounsaturates:* This group is believed to have none or very low cholesterol. Includes olive, canola, and peanut oils. Monounsaturates are also found in avocados, olives and most nuts.

The body needs a certain amount of fat but Americans get far too much of it in their diet. It is recommended that no more than 30 percent of your daily food intake should consist of fat. I figure that anything that hardens at room temperature is going to harden in my arteries.

# Chapter 23

# Foods for All Seasons

In the fall and winter, the body requires more calories for warmth just to perform regular tasks. In the spring and summer the living is easier and we don't need as many calories.

Wise Mother Nature must have had all this in mind when she shaped her food production and created the necessary foods for each season. Our ancestors planted corn, potatoes, onions, and legumes for winter storage and ate fresh fruits and vegetables that ripened in the spring and summer. They ate foods in their natural state and lived a life that was natural to them. Then came the processors, refiners, canners, and packagers with huge advertising budgets and we began to eat the same things all year round.

Somehow Mother Nature's scheme got lost in midwinter and we ate canned meats, canned vegetables, canned soups, macaroni and cheese, and cake mixes out of a box. In midsummer, when fruits and vegetables are available in their sun-ripened best, we still loaded our plates with canned foods, french fried potatoes, hot dogs, and marshmallows. Along the way we learned about antacids, pep pills, sleeping pills, and other crutches. Because of the unnatural diet, lack of activity, and that pooped-out feeling, around that fiftieth birthday we accepted the brainwashing that we were over the hill.

Speaking of canned and processed foods, I am not intimating that they are all bad for you but it's the overconsumption of them. Apples are good for you but, as I said before, you wouldn't eat a hundred a day would you? Read the ingredients on the label to see what you are actually buying. Today more and more processors are becoming health conscious.

My wife, Elaine, was a real junk food junkie when I met her, living on Danish sweet rolls and chocolate donuts for breakfast. For lunch: candy bars and soft drinks from the vending machines. For dinner: a hot dog or a can of roast beef, a can of vegetables, and ice cream for dessert. We were both on ABC-TV in San Francisco, she in the afternoons from 4:30 to 6:00 on the "Les Malloy Show" and I in the mornings at 9:00. I used to watch her come into the office every morning with her cigarette and chocolate donuts. As she tells it, "I poo-pooed Jack's philosophy but after hearing countless LaLannisms like: 'Ten seconds on the lips and a lifetime on your hips,' 'Your waistline is your lifeline,' 'The food you eat today is walking and talking tomorrow,' 'Use or Lose,' I started thinking about my life, and the way I looked. I was 27 and I felt old. I quit smoking cold turkey and asked Jack to set out a program for me." She started out easy by broiling everything she used to fry. She began to eat fresh vegetables and fruits and cut out all white flour and white sugar products. She says, "Changes took place in my body within a month. My skin became smoother and tighter. I reshaped my body through exercise and diet and my eyesight became more acute, the blues were bluer and the greens were greener." I am sure that had something to do with quitting cigarettes. Smoking constricts the blood vessels of the eyes. That was over forty years ago and last year she finished her fourth and fifth books on nutrition. Today she is a living example of health and vitality.

No matter where you live you can get fresh fruit. There are oranges, bananas, and apples all year long. A baked apple seasoned with honey, cinnamon, and lemon makes a great dessert. Although we are able to get fresh fruits and vegetables year round, every fruit and vegetable has a growing season when it is more plentiful. Not only is it more plentiful but it's also less expensive and fresher because it is often grown locally.

The U.S. government recommends that we eat at least three or four servings of vegetables and two or three servings of fruits every day. Currently only 40 percent of Americans get only three a day of the five to seven recommended.

In the fall months try to eat more locally grown vegetables like squash, pumpkins, yams, sweet potatoes, and carrots (high in beta carotene, an antioxidant), along with artichokes, asparagus, green beans, and tomatoes.

In the spring and summer, try to eat more strawberries, melons, cherries, grapes, and pears as they turn their cycle. You will be getting concentrated minerals and vitamins in the best possible way, all from natural foods.

In the hot summer, picnic lunches can really be a catastrophe for your health and body. It's almost traditional to make an outdoor lunch featuring sandwiches of cold cuts, hamburgers, hot dogs, fried chicken, soft drinks, cakes, cookies, and ice cream. Instead, try a picnic lunch that will fill you up not out and one that you won't wear on your waistline. Substitute water-packed tuna or sardines, unsalted peanut butter and honey sandwiches, or fresh roasted turkey or chicken on whole grain bread. Add hard-boiled eggs, celery and carrot sticks, nuts (like raw cashews and walnuts in moderation), along with more fresh seasonal fruits like grapes, peaches, apricots, and melons. Instead of soft drinks try making a a big thermos of unsweetened pineapple juice mixed with orange juice with a touch of lemon for tang.

When fresh fruits and vegetables are at their prime, try a day now and then when you pass up solid foods and just eat fresh fruits like watermelon, honeydew, cantaloupe, casabas and fresh vegetable juices along with plenty of water and you will help cleanse and detoxify your system. You'll find that it's an energy booster with minimal calories. Elaine and I go on a one-day watermelon fast during the summer. Every time we feel hungry we eat a piece of watermelon. When dinner time, our special time every evening, rolls around we go to the movies and take our watermelon with us. We don't miss our dinner because the movie is an entertaining substitute.

# Chapter 24

# Positive Doing: Get Out of the Rut and Do Something

Remember the story of the two frogs, Mike and Ike? Ike had fallen into a deep wagon rut and was positive he couldn't get out until a huge farm wagon was going to run over him. To avoid being killed he made a mighty jump onto the bank and his life was saved. Mike couldn't believe it and asked him how he did it. Ike's answer was, "I had to!" Maybe your life can be saved before an emergency comes along and strikes you down. Now is the time to act, now is the time to do something.

In this book I've set out a simple plan to help rejuvenate your body and increase your energy and vitality. What good is it if you don't read it? What good is a Rolls-Royce if you don't drive it? What good is the Bible if you don't read it? What good is all the knowledge I have accumulated over the last sixty years if you don't follow it? You have to act. Positive thinking is great but give me a positive *doer* along with it. Now a lot of you are saying you don't have time. A successful person always has the time or makes time to get the job done. Now you can put this aside and tell yourself that you'll get around to it later or you can decide to start right now. So if you feel as if those wheels are rolling over you, put your positive thinking with your positive doing and climb out of your rut!

First test your poise and strength of character when you're eating in a fine restaurant. Picture yourself with me; we're seated and the waiter is here for your order.

A cocktail? One is all right, if that's your custom. That's at least 80 calories and if you don't particularly want it, pass. Many people today will have wine with their meal. If you want to cut down the calories, try half wine and half water.

The waiter brings on the bread and is suggesting an appetizer. Right here you can add up the calories if you don't watch it. Too many good eaters load up their bread with butter and make the mistake of nibbling on goodies while having two or three cocktails. They overeat at the beginning and then don't enjoy the main course. Instead, if you want an appetizer ask for some carrot sticks and crisp celery. If you enjoy bread limit yourself to one slice and ask the waiter to bring you some olive oil and crushed garlic in a dish. Dip your bread in this and *voilà!* you'll love it.

Soup? Most good restaurants have a selection of at least two. Personally I love soup. The secret is to choose the one that is the least fattening. Instead of the fancy creamed soups ask for the ones lacking butter and cream.

Salad? Too many restaurants pass off the salad with a token of iceberg lettuce and a few tomato wedges. I ask the waiter or the manager to have the chef finely chop up five to ten of the raw vegetables they have in the kitchen, everything from green peppers to raw mushrooms. Even though they are chopped fine, chew them thoroughly and choose a low-calorie dressing. You can have a low-calorie salad and ruin it all with the hidden enemy, hundreds of calories of dressing. Ask for your dressing on the side, dip your fork into it and then take a bite of your salad. That little bit on the fork goes a long way. Here's another tip: The slower you eat, the less you will eat. Fast eaters always eat more.

The entree? The simpler the better. Sauces usually contain more calories. Broiled fish, chicken (try not to eat the skin as it is very high in calories), lean steak, pasta or a stir fry are good choices. With the entree, perhaps a baked potato but pass on the sour cream. Elaine often asks for just chives and puts a little of her garlic and oil on the potato. I scoop out the insides and eat the skins. But I often ask for rice instead of the potato. As for vegetables, most restaurants today will serve vegetables that are in season because they are cheaper and fresher. They also try to undercook them so they are crisp when you bite into them.

One more little hint. Don't salt and pepper your food before you taste it, it's a bad habit and an insult to the chef. That is one of my pet peeves.

Dessert? If you can skip it you are way ahead of the game but if you must have a dessert, how about some fresh fruit in season? If you are an ice cream eater, why not substitute nonfat frozen yogurt or sherbet?

Coffee and tea? Oh yes, I almost forgot about that because I never drink them. A wonderful substitute for those who want to cut down on coffee and tea is the large selection of herbal teas that are now readily available in most good restaurants. Try them all until you find the one you like. Elaine sometimes mixes two of them together. If you do drink either decaffeinated or regular coffee, cut down the calories by drinking it black and see that you get extra vitamin E, since vitamin E is destroyed by the caffeine. (Tests were done on truck drivers who were known to be heavy coffee drinkers and they were found to be lacking in vitamin E.)

Now let's go out to a dinner party where the host and hostess pride themselves on the elegance of their cuisine. They assume you'll eat everything and you don't want to tell them you're trying to cut down. So what are you going to do?

This is a good time to exercise some of your self-discipline. Remember, no one can force you to eat something you don't want. A good host and hostess won't insist when you decline something politely. If you feel that you can't mention that you are watching your calorie intake, pass on something you don't want and eat more of what you should be eating. If it's a high-calorie dressing, quietly push it aside with your fork and eat more of the salad. If it's fried chicken, remove the fried skin; do the same with anything deep fried. The meat inside is nicely steamed and tender. If your hostess insists that you taste her favorite dessert, take a small portion and let it remain on your plate. Part of our program is to be so in command of our lives we can become comfortable in all situations and walks of society.

Proper nutrition with proper exercise is a prime requisite for a healthy life after 50. However undereating is just as great a problem in our society as overeating. You won't feel or look better if you starve yourself, which can leave your body vulnerable to a nutrition deficiency. Like a car, the body must have fuel to keep the engine running properly.

Some people, as they get older, tend to eat less than they should and turn to more dry cereals and overprocessed foods. Some get their calories from cocktails to lift them over the rough spots, others subsist on milk, pudding, and ice cream and don't realize the importance of the need for macronutrients, fresh fruits and vegetables, of which I have already spoken.

For all of us, the banana offers a wealth of special health aids. It will satisfy your desire for something sweet and it's high in potassium and other minerals. It is highly digestible and is relatively low in calories. An average small banana contains about 80 calories and about one-third of man's RDA (recommended daily allowance) for vitamin C. The banana also helps to neutralize hydrochloric acid in the stomach and provide easily digestible protein. There is really no preparation involved; just peel and eat. As I mentioned earlier, try mashing a banana with a fork to release all the natural oils. This accentuates the sweet banana flavor, and your taste buds will dance with delight because they think they are eating a high-calorie pudding. Make sure the bananas are ripe. I like them when they have speckles on the skin; they tend to be a little sweeter.

Don't forget to read the labels on the food packages you buy. The Pure Food and Drug Act was set up to protect you and me. It helps to protect us against artificial colors and impurities. By reading labels, you will see the ingredients. The ingredients are listed in descending order by weight.

Not everyone approaching, or over 50, is overweight. Al Markstein, my high school buddy, who was not only born on the very same day as I, but even entered the Navy with me, recently found himself 20 pounds underweight. I suggested he start working out again and get on a good program of vitamins, minerals, and nutrition, increasing his caloric intake to 3,000 to 4,000 calories a day. (It takes 3,500 calories to gain a pound.) He made certain dietary changes and found a gym in his area that gave him personal supervision. Within months he not only gained back his 20 pounds, but his mental outlook improved and he doubled both his strength and his energy. He told me his friends are amazed at how great he looks and that he is doing things he hasn't been able to do in twenty-five years. This is an 80-year-old man who became a positive doer, proving that age doesn't matter and that it's never too late. If you are underweight, increase your caloric intake and get on a good exercise program. If you are overweight, decrease your caloric intake and get on a good exercise program. Exercise is a body normalizer.

## Chapter 25

# Create a Design for Living: Learn How to Play

Building health and vitality after 50 is to guarantee that your senior years will be just as active and full of fun as your youth, early adulthood, and middle years. People can and do live longer when they feel like living. Too many individuals scrimp and save for retirement but they neglect their health. When they are ready to retire they become ill and never reap the benefits of retirement. This happened to a very dear friend of ours who was always going to get started on a an exercise and nutrition program but it was always *mañana*. She retired at 65 and just a few months later suffered a stroke.

Too many have planned for retirement financially, but have forgotten to create a design for living. They've created a picture of themselves as old. If you think you're old, you're going to feel old. These people need to be revitalized with proper nutrition and regular exercise to get their lives in gear and forget about the "good old days." Now is the time to create your design for living and establish the health habits to carry you bouncing into your retirement years. Plenty of people do bounce after middle age. Just look around and you'll see a lot of them having more fun than kids and there's a reason for this. They're living, they're alive and vital. The old days were good but today is better. They're working at living not dying.

If we simply sit and let our bodies go to pot that is when the atrophy of unused muscles will show up. We can stop that accelerated aging process with a few simple exercises every day. You say it can't be done! Well, I just gave you an example in the previous chapter of my buddy Al who at 80 doubled his strength and doubled his energy.

I wish everyone could have seen the Public Broadcasting Service (PBS) production "The Challenge Within," part of the *The Infinite Voyage* series produced by WQED-TV, Pittsburgh, in conjunction with the National Academy of Sciences. It encompassed every facet of human endeavor, proving that anything is possible with the human body. In the segment on aging, Dr. Bill Evans of Tufts University in Boston felt that if athletes can train with high intensity so can older adults. He took a number of people in their sixties and seventies and put them on a high-intensity weight training program, and in six to eight weeks they doubled their muscle mass, strength, and endurance. He feels as I do that your muscles never lose the ability to respond to training and it's never too late. I proved this over the years in my gym in Oakland.

Along the same line, in a report in The *New England Journal of Medicine*, fitness tests were done at the Hebrew Rehabilitation Center near Boston where the average age is 88. It was discovered that lifting weights helped nursing home residents in their eighties and nineties walk more quickly and climb stairs more easily. Some were able to exchange their walkers for canes after ten weeks of working out. "These results suggest that one becomes weak not because of age but because of lack of activity and that strength training can improve their quality of life at any age," experts said. "A lot of what we think of as aging is really underuse," said Dr. Maria Fiatarone, head of the physiology lab at the U.S. Department of Agriculture Human Nutrition Research Center at Tufts, who led the study. "If you can prevent a lot of those changes caused by underuse, you will not get nearly as frail." Dr. Fiatarone's study is a follow-up to the widely reported 1990 pilot study of residents at the Hebrew Rehabilitation Center. Hooray! This is what I've been preaching for over sixty years ever since I invented the first leg extension and pulley machines.

Start now to create your design for living and learn how to play. Mickey Mantle in his book *All My Octobers* said, "I played 18 years, but if I had gotten more rest, worked out more, lived a drier life, I might not have been injured as much. I didn't lose my enthusiasm for the game I just lost the ability to do the things I used to do." He also said, "Willie Mays was one of the players who took care of himself, who really understood his body. I can tell you the mind may play games but the body never lies."

Just as your muscles need to be challenged to improve, you also need to be challenged mentally. Mental exercise, along with physical exercise and a good program of nutrition, is a real pepper-upper. You can't separate the mind and the body. How can you be challenged mentally? Set goals for yourself but don't set them so high that they're too difficult and you give up. Say you have 50 pounds to lose, don't think of the Herculean task of losing 50 pounds, think of 5 pounds, then 5 more pounds, little short-term goals. Have your sights set for your ultimate purpose but take one step at a time. How would you get to the top of a 25-story building without an elevator? You'd start with the first step and then the next and before you know it you'd reach your objective. A journey of a 1,000 miles begins with the first step.

Don't let stagnation set in. Unlock the key to being peppy and active. Exercise! Start with some of the exercises I've shown you and make haste slowly. The happiest people I know are the ones who play and are active. They aren't special American athletes at anything but they participate and they don't go to bed at night wondering if their world will fall apart. They are healthy and vital and they plan to remain that way for life. Be willing to learn a new active sport. Get in the habit of a workout at least three times a week. Join a gym, buy some home equipment or find a personal trainer. If you have access to a pool, lake, or ocean, work out in the water. You don't have to be able to swim to do water exercises. Years ago Orthopedic Hospital in Los Angeles pioneered a swimming pool therapy called water gymnastics. At the time, Dr. Charles L. Lowman reported how water exercise was useful in treating patients recovering from heart attacks. The body, he pointed out, is twenty-two times lighter under water than out of it and it takes proportionately less effort to exercise. This allows heart patients to exercise in pools soon after attacks, and progress through easy stages to more kinds of exercises until they are walking and moving about normally. I started my Jack LaLanne Hydronastics, exercising in the pool, over sixty years ago and continue it to this day. Doesn't it stand to reason that if exercise is good for one after a heart attack, wouldn't it be better to start exercising *before* a heart attack? Just **Running in the Water** is a wonderful exercise to help firm up the thighs, hips, and midsection. Another exercise is **Arm Crosses in the Water**. Stand in water up to your chest and your arms straight out to the side. Now, with cupped hands, bring your arms around through the water in front of you until they cross, pulling hard against the water's resistance. Reverse and push your hands back around through the water to the original position. Push and pull. Cross and recross. This exercise helps firm the front of your chest, working those pectoral muscles. When you push back you're working your upper back. If you cannot swim, just stand in the water chest to neck high and do the **Crawl Stroke Exercise**. If you have access to as pool, hold on to the edge, face down, and **flutter kick** vigorously from your hips, breathe deeply, making big movements, keeping your legs straight. Great cardiovascular exercise for the waist, hips, thighs, and lower back. Now turn around so that your elbows are on the edge of the pool or in the gutter, pretend you are **pumping a bicycle**. Another great cardio-vascular exercise.

If you have never learned to swim, why not now? Or learn to dance. Western dancing seems to be all the rage now, so why not join a class, it will give you a lot of pleasure and wonderful exercise. Give bowling a try, ski, fish, and even Ping-Pong can be exerting. Travel, paint, or start a new career.

Another key to feeling peppy is nutrition. If you are putting live and vital food into your body you are going to feel live and vital. If you are putting lifeless, over-processed, overcooked junk food into your body you are going to feel lifeless. As I've said before, everything works for the body mentally and physically. Negative thoughts lead to a negative reaction to the body, positive thoughts lead to a positive reaction. For every action there is a reaction. It's like planting seeds. If you plant alfalfa, alfalfa comes up, if you plant poison ivy, poison ivy comes up. Remember, every food you eat has an action on the body either positive or negative. You are the planter, the farmer of your body, it's your choice to put in good or bad foods.

I have already mentioned that the U.S. government recommends at least five to seven servings of fruits and vegetables every day. Make this one of your goals and try to select fresh fruits and vegetables. Eating cruciferous vegetables may help prevent some cancers. They include cabbage, broccoli, brussel sprouts, cauliflower, and kohlrabi. There is also some evidence to suggest that garlic and onion may help to bring down blood pressure. Green and yellow vegetables, such as carrots, winter squash, pumpkins, sweet potatoes, spinach and broccoli, and yellow fruits help replenish vitamin A. Potatoes that aren't loaded with sour cream, cheese, or butter are a low-calorie source of complex carbohydrates and potassium. Cook brown rice instead of white rice. Pass on the organ meats because of their high cholesterol content. Among red meats "choice" and "prime" contain more saturated fats. Leaner cuts are labeled "select." Fish, such as salmon, cod, and halibut, are rich in cholesterol-lowering omega-3 fatty acids. Shellfish like crab and shrimp are high in cholesterol. Poultry is better cooked without the skin; leaving the skin on will push up the fat content. If you do cook the chicken with the skin on, remove it before eating. The white meat has less fat than the dark meat. Most luncheon meats are high in fat calories. Turkey, ham, or turkey bologna may derive 30 to 50 percent of their calories from fat. Herbs are useful seasoning in place of salt. Include more protein-rich dried beans and peas, peanut butter, tofu, and, in moderation, eggs. As I explained earlier, the white of the egg contains approximately 15 calories whereas the whole egg contains about 70. Select whole grain breads instead of white. Don't let the name of the bread mislead you. The first ingredient printed on the label is the main ingredient. Color is no indicator of bread nutrition. Raisin juice or molasses may have been added. Vegetable oils have no cholesterol, but watch for coconut or palm oil in some of your bakery goods. These oils are high in saturated fatty acids that encourage the body to produce more cholesterol. If you are going to drink milk for your calcium, drink skim milk because it contains less than 0.5 percent of its calories from fat, whereas 2 percent milk derives 38 percent of its calories from fat. Choose nonfat yogurt instead of sour cream. Tofu can provide protein as well as calcium. As for cheeses, stick with the low-salt, low-fat types like string, mozzarella, and low-fat ricotta. Eat a bagel but skip the cream cheese, which is about 90 percent fat. Crackers and cookies and other snacks can add lots of fat and sugar to your diet. Choose sorbet, fruit ices, and sherbets instead of ice cream. The National Research Council, Food and Nutrition Board, recommends a range of 1,400 to 2,200 calories per day for females ages 51 to 75 and 2,000 to 2,800 for men. For those who are older than 75, 1,200 to 2,000 for women, and 1,650 to 2,400 for men.

When you are exercising and eating properly, everything gets better, even your sex life. A 50-year-old whose blood sugar drops tends to lose all drives, the sex drive among them. The act of love demands energy and vigor. (The last thing any tired person wants is sex.) It demands health, both mental and physical. Nutrition revitalizes and exercise builds energy.

"I don't know what my husband is doing down in that gym," a woman once wrote me. "He used to come home from work too pooped for romance. Now you're either going to have to slow him down or I'm going to have to come in to keep up with him." She actually came in to my women's department soon after. There wasn't any magic to what we did for the husband. We were doing precisely what I am urging you to do in this book. Through sound exercise and nutrition we were removing the signs of neglect. We were helping this man convince himself that he didn't need to look and feel old. It worked.

I have tried from the very first chapter to show you that what you must conquer is self-doubt, surrendering to old age, and lack of confidence. I've tried to show you how good health in a vital, energetic body can overcome most obstacles that come with the years. I can only go back to my first premise, that balanced meals, proper supplements, and exercise are the key to a healthy, happy lifestyle.

So there you are, judge for yourself. Go back to the mirror where this all started and see how you measure up. Start at the bottom and work your way up. Could you stand to lose a few pounds? Is your wardrobe up to date? What about your hair, does it make you look younger? As you look at your reflection do these things make you smile? If not, smile anyway because this is the first day of the rest of your life and "anything in life is possible!"

Remember, age is a state of mind. I urge you to work on yours now.

# Chapter 26

# Sculpturing the New You

Now that you have acquired new habits of proper exercise and nutrition, keep it up. Do not miss your workouts for any reason. If you miss one, it will be easy for you to miss the next, and before you know it you have broken the habit.

Being in condition means that every muscle in your body is getting its share of work. If any of the muscles are neglected you will not be able to achieve peak performance. You get out of life what you put into it. So it goes with exercising. If you exercise half-heartedly, so the results will be. If you put effort into your exercises, you will reap the rewards of health, happiness, strength, endurance, and a sound body. "Exercise for life, for the rest of your life," is my motto. The older we are the more we need it.

I have outlined a sample program to help assist you in making your own workouts. First of all I want you to take your measurements, in inches. Measure yourself from chest to ankle; then enter the results on your Progress Chart. Keep entering each week as you progress toward your final goal.

# Height and Weight Tables

## Men

| Height Feet | Inches | Small Frame | Medium Frame | Large Frame |
|---|---|---|---|---|
| 5 | 2 | 128-134 | 131-141 | 138-150 |
| 5 | 3 | 130-136 | 133-143 | 140-153 |
| 5 | 4 | 132-138 | 135-145 | 142-156 |
| 5 | 5 | 134-140 | 137-151 | 144-160 |
| 5 | 6 | 136-142 | 139-151 | 146-164 |
| 5 | 7 | 138-145 | 142-154 | 149-168 |
| 5 | 8 | 140-148 | 145-157 | 152-172 |
| 5 | 9 | 142-151 | 148-160 | 155-176 |
| 5 | 10 | 144-154 | 151-163 | 158-180 |
| 5 | 11 | 146-157 | 154-166 | 161-184 |
| 6 | 0 | 149-160 | 157-170 | 164-188 |
| 6 | 1 | 152-164 | 160-174 | 168-192 |
| 6 | 2 | 155-168 | 164-178 | 172-197 |
| 6 | 3 | 158-172 | 167-182 | 176-202 |
| 6 | 4 | 162-176 | 171-187 | 181-207 |

## Height and Weight Tables (*continued*)

### Women

| Height Feet Inches | | Small Frame | Medium Frame | Large Frame |
|---|---|---|---|---|
| 4 | 10 | 102-111 | 109-121 | 118-131 |
| 4 | 11 | 103-113 | 111-123 | 120-134 |
| 5 | 0 | 104-115 | 113-126 | 122-137 |
| 5 | 1 | 106-118 | 115-129 | 125-140 |
| 5 | 2 | 108-121 | 118-132 | 128-143 |
| 5 | 3 | 111-124 | 121-135 | 131-147 |
| 5 | 4 | 114-127 | 124-138 | 134-151 |
| 5 | 5 | 117-130 | 127-141 | 137-155 |
| 5 | 6 | 120-133 | 130-144 | 140-159 |
| 5 | 7 | 123-136 | 133-147 | 143-163 |
| 5 | 8 | 126-139 | 136-153 | 146-170 |
| 5 | 9 | 129-142 | 139-153 | 149-170 |
| 5 | 10 | 132-145 | 142-156 | 152-176 |
| 5 | 11 | 135-148 | 145-159 | 155-176 |
| 6 | 0 | 138-151 | 148-162 | 158-179 |

Weights at ages 25±59 based on lowest mortality. Weight in pounds according to frame (in indoor clothing weighing 5 lbs. for men and 3 lbs. for women; shoes with 1″ heels).

Source of basis data: 1979 Build Study. Society of Actuaries and Association of Life Insurance Medical Directors of America, 1980. Reprinted Courtesy of Metropolitan Life Insurance Company
© 1983 Metropolitan Life Insurance Company

Now let's refresh your memory on all the exercises I have given you.

## Exercise Chart

### Head, Face, and Neck

Chapter 12   Make Faces
            Smile
            Scalp Massage
            Chin on Chest
            Head Raises

### Shoulders

Chapter 5    Swimming
Chapter 10   Shoulder Shrugs
Chapter 11   Two-way Punches
            Swings
Chapter 13   Door-Frame Stretch
Chapter 16   Arm Raises to Front
            Military Press
            Taut Towel
Chapter 25   Crawl Stroke in Water

### Chest

Chapter 5    Chair Push-ups
            Wall Push-ups
            Pullovers
Chapter 11   Two-way Punches
Chapter 13   Door-Frame Stretch
Chapter 25   Arm Crosses in Water

### Arms and Hands

Chapter 10   Biceps Curls
            Triceps Extensions
Chapter 16   Open and Close Hands
            Newspaper Roll

Rubber Ball Squeeze
Arm Raises to Front
Arm Raises to Sides
Military Press

## Upper Back

Chapter 2      Ceiling Stretch
Chapter 10     Bent Over Rows
Chapter 16     Parallel Towel
               Military Press
Chapter 25     Arm Crosses in Water
               Crawl Stroke in Water

## Lower Back

Chapter 2      Side to Side Stretch
               Through the Legs Stretch
Chapter 5      Flutter Kick on armless chair
Chapter 10     Bend Over Stretch
Chapter 11     Swings
               Leg Extensions to the Back
Chapter 14     Cat Stretch
               One Arm Dead Lift

## Waist and Abdomen

Chapter 2      Side to Side Stretch
Chapter 3      Straight Leg Lifts
Chapter 11     Swings
               Knees to Chest
Chapter 13     Stretch to Backbone
               Waist Away from Belt
Chapter 14     Knees to Chest
               Crunches
               Side Bends
Chapter 16     Leg Lifts with Book

## Hips and Thighs

## Lower Legs and Feet

## Cardiovascular

## Posture

## All-Over Exercises

Chapter 2      Bed Stretches
Chapter 10     Windmill
               Get-up and Get-downs
Chapter 11     Swings

I have included a sample workout program, using the exercises listed above, for you to refer to when making your own program. Concentrate on your problem zones. Do exercises that you have never done before. Feel free to use this sample but also make up your own workouts to fit your own needs. And be sure to change your program every two to three weeks. The muscles respond only when they are challenged beyond what they are used to doing.

# Week of

| Exercise | Date / Reps | | | | | | | |
|---|---|---|---|---|---|---|---|---|

### Head, Face and Neck

| Exercise | 1 | 2 | 3 | 4 | 5 | 6 | 7 | 8 |
|---|---|---|---|---|---|---|---|---|
| Chin on Chest | 2 / 10 | | | | 1-5 / 10 | | 1-7 / 10 | 1-8 / 10 |
| Head Raises | | 1-3 / 5 | | | | 1-6 / 10 | | |

### Shoulders

| Exercise | 1 | 2 | 3 | 4 | 5 | 6 | 7 | 8 |
|---|---|---|---|---|---|---|---|---|
| Shoulder Shrugs | 1-2 / 20 | | | 1-4 / 15 | | 1-6 / 20 | 1-7 / 20 | |
| Military Press | | 1-3 / 10 | | | 1-5 / 10 | 1-6 / 10 | | 1-8 / 10 |

### Chest

| Exercise | 1 | 2 | 3 | 4 | 5 | 6 | 7 | 8 |
|---|---|---|---|---|---|---|---|---|
| Chair Push-ups | | 1-3 / 5 | 1-4 / 5 | 1-5 / 10 | | | | 1-8 / 10 |
| Arm Crosses | 1-2 / 25 | | 1-4 / 20 | | | 1-6 / 20 | 1-7 / 20 | |

### Arms and Hands

| Exercise | 1 | 2 | 3 | 4 | 5 | 6 | 7 | 8 |
|---|---|---|---|---|---|---|---|---|
| Biceps Curls | | 1-3 / 20 | | | 1-5 / 20 | 1-6 / 20 | | |
| Newspaper Roll | 1-2 / 15 | | | 1-4 / 15 | | | 1-7 / 15 | 1-8 / 20 |

### Upper Back

| Exercise | 1 | 2 | 3 | 4 | 5 | 6 | 7 | 8 |
|---|---|---|---|---|---|---|---|---|
| Parallel Towel | 1-2 / 10 | | | 1-4 / 10 | | | | 1-8 / 20 |
| Ceiling Stretch | 1-2 / 10 sec | | | | 1-5 / 20 sec | 1-6 / 20 sec | 1-7 / 30 sec | |

## Lower Back

| Exercise | | | | | | | | |
|---|---|---|---|---|---|---|---|---|
| Bend Over Stretch | | 1-3 / 10 sec | 1-4 / 10 sec | | 1-6 / 15 sec | | | 1-8 / 15 sec |
| One Arm Dead Lift | 1-2 / 10 | | 1-4 / 10 | 1-5 / 15 | | | 1-7 / 15 | |

## Waist and Abdomen

| Exercise | | | | | | | | |
|---|---|---|---|---|---|---|---|---|
| Side to Side Stretch | | 1-3 / 20 | | | 1-5 / 20 | | 1-7 / 20 | 1-8 / 20 |
| Crunches | 1-2 / 15 | | | 1-4 / 15 | | 1-6 / 15 | | |

## Hips and Thighs

| Exercise | | | | | | | | |
|---|---|---|---|---|---|---|---|---|
| Hamstring Stretch | 1-2 / 5 | | | | 1-5 / 5 | 1-6 / 10 | | |
| Leg Ext. to Back | | 1-3 / 20 | 1-4 / 20 | | | | 1-7 / 20 | 1-8 / 25 |

## Lower Legs and Feet

| Exercise | | | | | | | | |
|---|---|---|---|---|---|---|---|---|
| Toe Raises | | 1-3 / 10 | 1-4 / 10 | 1-5 / 15 | | | | 1-8 / 15 |
| Self-Resisting Leg Ext | 1-2 / 5 | | | | | 1-6 / 10 | 1-7 / 10 | |

## Cardiovascular

| Exercise | | | | | | | | |
|---|---|---|---|---|---|---|---|---|
| Two-Way Punches | | 1-3 / 40 | | | 1-6 / 40 | | | 1-8 / 40 |
| Windmill | 1-2 / 5 | | 1-4 / 10 | 1-5 / 10 | | 1-7 / 15 | | |

## Posture

| Exercise | | | | | | | | |
|---|---|---|---|---|---|---|---|---|
| Swimming | | 1-3 / 30 | | 1-5 / 30 | | 1-7 / 30 | | |
| Tiger Stretch | 1-2 / 10 | | 1-4 / 10 | | 1-6 / 10 | | 1-8 / 10 | |

Now use this page to make up your own program.

## Week of

**Exercise** Date / Reps

**Head, Face and Neck**

**Shoulders**

**Chest**

**Arms and Hands**

**Upper Back**

**Lower Back**

**Waist and Abdomen**

**Hips and Thighs**

**Lower Legs and Feet**

**Cardiovascular**

**Posture**